The Atlas of Heart Disease and Stroke

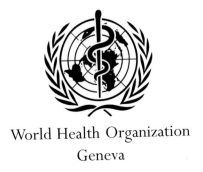

World Health Organization

Geneva

In the same series:

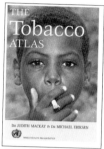

The Tobacco Atlas

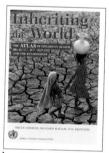

Inheriting the World:
The Atlas of Children's Health and the Environment

The Atlas of Heart Disease and Stroke

Dr Judith Mackay and Dr George A. Mensah

with

Dr Shanthi Mendis and Dr Kurt Greenlund

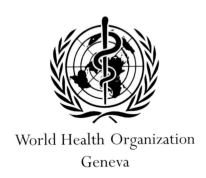

World Health Organization

Geneva

The Atlas of Heart Disease and Stroke © World Health Organization 2004

First published 2004
1 3 5 7 9 10 8 6 4 2

WHO Library Cataloguing-in-Publication Data
Mackay, Judith.
The atlas of heart disease and stroke / Judith Mackay and George Mensah;
with Shanthi Mendis and Kurt Greenlund.
1.Heart diseases – epidemiology 2.Cerebrovascular accident – epidemiology
3.Risk factors 4.Atlases I.Mensah, George. II.Mendis, Shanthi.
III.Greenlund, Kurt. IV.Title.

ISBN 92 4 156276 8
(NLM Classification: WG 210)

Produced for the World Health Organization by
Myriad Editions Limited
6–7 Old Steine, Brighton BN1 1EJ, UK
http://www.MyriadEditions.com

Coordinated for Myriad Editions by Candida Lacey
Edited by Hayley Ann
Design and graphics by Corinne Pearlman
Maps created by Isabelle Lewis

Publications of the World Health Organization can be obtained from:
Marketing and Dissemination, World Health Organization, 20 Avenue Appia, 1211 Geneva 27, Switzerland
tel: +41 22 791 2476; fax: +41 22 791 4857; email: bookorders@who.int
Requests for permission to reproduce or translate WHO publications,
whether for sale or for noncommercial distribution,
should be addressed to Publications, at the above address
fax: +41 22 791 4806; email: permissions@who.int

Printed and bound in Hong Kong, China
Produced through Phoenix Offset Limited under the supervision of Bob Cassels, The Hanway Press, London

Contents

Foreword

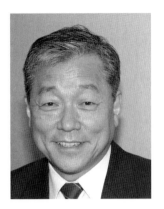

A message from

Dr LEE Jong-Wook
Director-General
World Health Organization

Heart disease and stroke are currently the leading cause of death in all developed countries and in most developing countries. There were approximately 17 million deaths due to cardiovascular disease in 2003 – one-third of all deaths in the world.

It is disturbing to note that at least 75% of deaths from heart disease and stroke now occur in the poorer regions of the world, which also face major threats from communicable diseases. These regions thus suffer under the so-called "double burden" of disease. If preventive action is not taken urgently, heart disease and stroke – which are already major public health problems – will rapidly advance across regions and social classes to reach epidemic proportions worldwide.

We know that the major risk factors for heart disease and stroke are high blood pressure, high blood cholesterol, tobacco use, physical inactivity, unhealthy diet and obesity. Many of these risk factors result from unhealthy lifestyles. These unhealthy lifestyle habits, which are linked to urbanization, often start in childhood and youth, encouraged by the influence of mass advertising and social pressures. This underscores the importance of targeting children and young people in all programmes that aim to prevent heart disease and stroke.

Prevention and control of heart disease and stroke in developing countries represent a challenging task. There are a number of major barriers to progress, including lack of reliable epidemiological information, inaccessibility of health care, shortages of trained manpower and resources, and misconceptions about heart disease and stroke among policy-makers and the public.

However, the good news is that knowledge about the causes of heart disease and stroke is growing, and various countries are gaining experience in translating this knowledge into effective action.

I believe that our efforts to control heart disease and stroke can only succeed if they are focused at country level. Current WHO activities in this area are based on the WHO Global Strategy for the Prevention and Control of Noncommunicable Disease, which was adopted by the World Health Assembly in 2000. Our goals are to:

- provide guidance to countries on policy, legislative and financial measures that can help prevent cardiovascular disease;
- assess and track the magnitude of the cardiovascular disease epidemic and its social, economic, behavioural and political determinants in developing countries;
- reduce cardiovascular risk factors and their determinants and promote cardiovascular health for all age groups;
- strengthen the health care of people with cardiovascular disease by developing norms and guidelines for cost-effective interventions.

To achieve these goals, WHO has developed standardized approaches to strengthen national surveillance systems for key risk factors. Further, WHO has initiated programmes at country level to scale up health care for those with established cardiovascular disease and to introduce affordable and innovative approaches for managing cardiovascular risk factors and cardiovascular disease in low-resource settings.

WHO is also in the process of addressing some of the main risk factors for cardiovascular disease through global action, such as the Framework Convention on Tobacco Control and the Global Strategy on Diet, Physical Activity and Health. These strategies will help countries in their efforts to develop and implement policies to reduce the burden of cardiovascular disease.

We recognize that advocacy, resource mobilization, capacity development, and research are necessary to galvanize global action against the causes of cardiovascular disease. WHO is working with other UN agencies, research institutions, nongovernmental organizations, the private sector and civil society to promote these activities. Together, we can move the global public health agenda forward to avert unnecessary deaths and suffering due to this eminently preventable disease.

Preface

"We have the scientific knowledge to create a world
in which most heart disease and stroke could be eliminated."
The Victoria Declaration on Heart Health, 1992

"Change before you have to."
Jack Welch,
former Chairman and Chief Executive Officer of
General Electric, USA (1935–)

Heart disease and stroke, the main cardiovascular diseases, are truly global epidemics. They deserve the attention of governments, policy-makers, national and international organizations, committed individuals and families everywhere.

Heart disease and stroke are no longer diseases of old men in developed countries. They are also diseases of women, young adults, and even children. They affect the wealthy and the poor. Already they claim more lives in developing than developed countries. The Asian girl on the cover is at risk, as are many children and young adults throughout the world.

The risk factors for heart disease and stroke begin in youth, and most can be prevented or controlled. Yet, worldwide, most people who have risk factors are either not treated or are inadequately treated. Special attention to high blood pressure, high blood cholesterol, tobacco and other major risk factors is crucial.

Cardiovascular diseases are more than just health problems: both the diseases and their underlying causes have major financial implications for governments, businesses and individuals. The "globesity" epidemic is causing international concern. The tobacco epidemic is linked to smuggling, big business and politics. If people are to be encouraged to take regular physical activity, commitment is needed from both individuals and society. The prevention and control of high blood pressure and high blood cholesterol require action from governments and the pharmaceutical industry, not just individual patients.

Research achievements in the field of heart disease and stroke have been phenomenal. We know a lot today, but as Goethe put it, "knowing is not enough, we must apply." We must apply what we already know, and translate the best science into practice for the benefit of all, worldwide.

The good news, as stated most eloquently in the Victoria Declaration on Heart Health more than a decade ago, is that we know what we need to do to eliminate most heart disease and stroke. What is needed now is the combination of necessary resources and political will on a global scale to take effective action. Now is the time to act – and to change before we have to.

Judith Mackay, Hong Kong SAR, China
George A. Mensah, Atlanta, GA, USA

Acknowledgements

Special thanks go to the following WHO staff for their support for this project: Catherine Le Galès-Camus, Assistant Director-General, Noncommunicable Diseases and Mental Health; Robert Beaglehole, Director, Department of Chronic Diseases and Health Promotion; Rafael Bengoa, Director, Health Systems Policy and Operations; and Derek Yach, Representative of the Director-General.

Particular thanks go to the Centers for Disease Control and Prevention (CDC), United States of America, for their generous financial support of this atlas.

For their creativity, artistic talent and innovative suggestions in the design and cartography of this atlas, we would like to thank the Myriad Editions team of Candida Lacey, Corinne Pearlman, Hayley Ann and Isabelle Lewis.

Sincere thanks go to Pat Butler for her editorial input, and to all colleagues at the World Health Organization:

Dele Abegunde, Technical Officer, Cardiovascular Diseases, Noncommunicable Diseases and Mental Health;

Timothy Armstrong, Technical Officer, Surveillance and Information for Policy, Noncommunicable Diseases and Mental Health;

Vishal Arora, Noncommunicable Diseases and Mental Health, South East Asia Region (SEARO);

Fabienne Besson, Secretary, Management of Noncommunicable Diseases, Noncommunicable Diseases and Mental Health;

Ties Boerma, Director, Measurement and Health Information Systems, Evidence and Information for Policy;

Ruth Bonita, Director, Surveillance, Office of Assistant Director-General, Evidence and Information for Policy;

Gian Luca Burci, Senior Legal Officer, Office of the Legal Counsel;

Somnath Chatterji, Scientist, Classification, Assessment, Surveys and Terminology, Evidence and Information for Policy;

Charles Gollmar, Group Leader, School Health and Youth Health Promotion, Noncommunicable Diseases and Mental Health;

Carina Marquez, Technical Officer, Surveillance and Information for Policy, Noncommunicable Diseases and Mental Health;

Colin Mathers, Scientist, Epidemiology and Burden of Disease, Evidence and Information for Policy;

Shanthi Mendis, Coordinator, Cardiovascular Diseases, Noncommunicable Diseases and Mental Health;

Patricia Mucavele, Technical Officer, Nutrition for Health and Development, Noncommunicable Diseases and Mental Health;

Mona Nassef, Secretary, Cardiovascular Diseases, Noncommunicable Diseases and Mental Health;

Chizuru Nishida, Scientist, Nutrition for Health and Development, Noncommunicable Diseases and Mental Health;

Tomoko Ono, Technical Officer, Surveillance and Information for Policy, Noncommunicable Diseases and Mental Health;

Leanne Riley, Scientist, School Health and Youth Health Promotion, Noncommunicable Diseases and Mental Health;

Gojka Roglic, Technical Officer, Diabetes Mellitus, Noncommunicable Diseases and Mental Health;

Jukka Sailas, Scientist, Management Support Unit, Evidence and Information for Policy, Noncommunicable Diseases and Mental Health;

Bakuti Shengelia, Medical Officer, Cardiovascular Diseases, Noncommunicable Diseases and Mental Health;

Kate Strong, Acting Team Coordinator, Surveillance and Information for Policy, Noncommunicable Diseases and Mental Health;

Bedirhan Ustun, Coordinator, Classification, Assessment, Surveys and Terminology, Evidence and Information for Policy;

Pierre-Michel Virot, Audiovisual and Training Team, Information Technology and Telecommunications;

Amalia Waxman, Project Manager, Noncommunicable Diseases and Mental Health.

Thanks to our colleagues at the National Center for Chronic Disease Prevention and Health Promotion, Centers for Disease Control and Prevention (CDC), United States of America:

Laurie D. Elam-Evans, Deputy Associate Director for Science, Division of Adult and Community Health;

Wayne H. Giles, Associate Director of Science, Division of Adult and Community Health;

Kurt J. Greenlund, Senior Epidemiologist, Science and Communication Unit, Cardiovascular Health

Branch, Division of Adult and Community Health;

Mary E. Hall, Public Health Analyst, Office of the Director;

Virginia Bales Harris, Director, Division of Adult and Community Health;

Marsha L. Houston, Health Communication Specialist, Cardiovascular Health Branch, Division of Adult and Community Health;

Frederick L. Hull, Deputy Chief, Technical Information and Editorial Services Branch, Office of the Director;

Margaret Malone, Deputy Chief, Cardiovascular Health Branch, Division of Adult and Community Health;

James S. Marks, Director.

For their input on particular maps and subjects, we would like to thank the following:

4 Risk factors start in childhood and youth
Samira Asma, Associate Director, Global Tobacco Control, Office on Smoking and Health, Centers for Disease Control and Prevention, USA; Jonathan R. Carapetis, Consultant in Paediatric Infectious Diseases, Centre for International Child Health, University of Melbourne, Australia; Gilles Paradis, Division of Preventive Medicine, McGill University Health Center, Montreal, Canada; Neville Rigby, Director of Policy and Public Affairs, International Obesity TaskForce, International Association for the Study of Obesity; Charles W. Warren, Distinguished Consultant /Demographer, Global Tobacco Control, Office on Smoking and Health, Centers for Disease Control and Prevention, USA.

5 Risk factor: blood pressure Yussuf Saloojee, tobacco control advocate, South Africa.

6 Risk factor: lipids Robert Clarke, Clinical Trial Service Unit, Oxford University, United Kingdom; Rory Collins, Clinical Trial Service Unit, Oxford University, United Kingdom.

7 Risk factor: tobacco Omar Shafey, Manager, International Tobacco Surveillance, American Cancer Society, USA.

8 Risk factor: physical inactivity Krishnan Anand, Associate Professor, Centre for Community Medicine, All India Institute of Medical Sciences, India.

12 Women: a special case? Sandra Coney, women's health advocate, New Zealand.

18 Research Rory Collins, Clinical Trial Service Unit, Oxford University, United Kingdom; Hugh Tunstall-Pedoe, Cardiovascular Epidemiology Unit, University of Dundee, United Kingdom (MONICA study).

19 Organizations *Children's Heart Link (USA)*: Karen Baumgaertner, International Programs Associate; John Cushing, International Programs Director. *International Association for the Study of Obesity*: Neville Rigby, Director of Policy and Public Affairs, International Obesity TaskForce. *International Stroke Society*: Julien Bogousslavsky, President-Elect; Frank M. Yatsu, Treasurer. *World Heart Federation*: Carola Adler, World Heart Day Manager; Sara Bowen, Website/IT Manager; Sania Nishtar, Chairman, World Heart Day Committee; Philip Poole-Wilson, President; Janet Voûte, Chief Executive Officer.

22 Health education *World Heart Federation* (as above); Eeva Riitta Vartiainen, Project Manager, International Quit and Win, Finland.

23 Policies and legislation Omar Shafey, Manager, International Tobacco Surveillance, American Cancer Society, USA.

25 The future Rory Collins, Clinical Trial Service Unit, Oxford University, United Kingdom; Anthony Rodgers, Clinical Trials Research Unit, University of Auckland, New Zealand.

26 Chronology Julien Bogousslavsky, President-Elect, International Stroke Society; Rory Collins, Clinical Trial Service Unit, Oxford University, United Kingdom; John W. Farquhar, Stanford Prevention Research Center, USA; David Simpson, International Agency on Tobacco and Health, London, United Kingdom.

We are also extremely grateful to our families for their support during the preparation of this atlas.

For the use of photographs, we would like to thank the following:
Front cover Amy, Hong Kong © Guy Nowell, Hong Kong SAR, China. http://www.guynowell.com
Back cover photographs Cardiology operation, Mauritius © WHO/Harry Anenden; man selling vegetables, India © WHO/Pierre Virot; man on bench © iStock/Tomaz Levstek; Woman and girl buying sweets, India © WHO/Pierre Virot
Part 1 Child health examination, Cuba © WHO/Carlos Gaggero
Part 2 Woman cooking, Guatemala © WHO/Armando Waak

Part 3 Cardiology operation, USA © WHO/Jean Mohr

Part 4 Youth sport, Germany © WHO/Tibor Farkas

Part 5 Adolescent group, Peru © WHO/Julio Vizcarra

Part 6 Man selling vegetables, India © WHO/Pierre Virot

1 Types of cardiovascular disease Heart © Hemera Photo-Objects

4 Risk factors start in childhood and youth Boy smoking, Seychelles © WHO/Harry Anenden; burger © Hemera Photo-Objects

6 Risk factor: lipids Arteries © American Heart Association; rice bowl © Hemera Photo-Objects

7 Risk factor: tobacco Smoking hand; young people, Canada © WHO/J L Ray; road signs, USA © Corinne Pearlman

8 Risk factor: physical inactivity TV viewer, biker, wheelchair user, woman with push-chair © Hemera Photo-Objects; people on scooter, New Delhi © Candida Lacey

9 Risk factor: obesity Groceries, USA © USDA/Ken Hammond; apple and pear © Woodrow Phoenix/Comic Company/British Dietetic Association

10 Risk factor: diabetes Men playing basketball, Finland © WHO/Farkas Tibor

11 Risk factor: socioeconomic status Young boy smoking, China © Carol Betson

12 Women: a special case? Hospital patient, Finland © WHO/Tibor Farkas; smoking woman © iStock/Tan Kian Khoon; obese woman © iStock/Annette Birkenfeld; women walking © iStock/Leah-Anne Thompson; menopausal woman © iStock/Joseph Jean Rolland Dubé

13 Global burden of coronary heart disease Cardiology operation, Mauritius © WHO/Harry Anenden

14 Deaths from coronary heart disease Cardiology operation, USA © WHO/Jean Mohr; heart © Hemera Photo-Objects

15 Global burden of stroke Pills © iStock/Amanda Rohde

16 Deaths from stroke Man on bench © iStock/Tomaz Levstek

17 Economic costs Rice © USDA/Ken Hammond; potatoes © USDA/Ken Hammond

19 Organizations WHO HQ Geneva © WHO/Pierre Virot

20 Prevention: personal choices and actions Salad, USA © Corinne Pearlman; Amy, Hong Kong © Guy Nowell; grapefruit, runner © Hemera Photo-Objects

21 Prevention: population and systems approaches Good Heart Food leaflet © British Dietetic Association/Comic Company; hospital computer, UK © WHO/P Larsen; health examination © WHO/Julio Vizcarra

22 Health Education Posters © World Heart Federation

23 Policies and legislation Singapore bus © WHO/Tibor Farkas; display, gymnasium, Singapore, © WHO; fried food, USA (bar chart) © Corinne Pearlman; man smoking, Sri Lanka (bar chart) © Garrett Mehl; burger © Hemera Photo-Objects

24 Treatment Man on bike, Finland © WHO/Tibor Farkas

25 The future Woman, Rwanda © WHO/J. L. Ray

Whilst every reasonable effort has been made to contact the copyright holders of images used in the atlas, the authors and publisher will gladly receive information that will enable them to rectify any inadvertent errors in subsequent editions.

About the authors

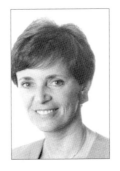

Dr Judith Mackay
MBChB, FRCP (Edin), FRCP (Eng)

Dr Judith Mackay is a medical doctor based in Hong Kong Special Administrative Region, China, and a Senior Policy Adviser to the World Health Organization. After an early career as a hospital physician, she became a health advocate. She is a Fellow of the Royal Colleges of Physicians of Edinburgh and of London, and an Honorary Fellow of the Hong Kong College of Cardiology. Dr Mackay has received many international awards, including the WHO Commemorative Medal, the Fries Prize for Improving Health, the Luther Terry Award for Outstanding Individual Leadership, the International Partnering for World Health Award, and the Founding International Achievement Award from the Asia Pacific Association for the Control of Tobacco. She is the author of *The Tobacco Atlas, The State of Health Atlas* and *The Penguin Atlas of Human Sexual Behavior*.

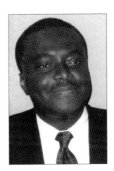

Dr George A. Mensah
MD, FACC, FACP, FESC

Dr George Mensah is acting director, the National Center for Chronic Disease Prevention and Health Promotion, and chief of the Cardiovascular Health Branch at the Centers for Disease Control and Prevention in Atlanta, Georgia, USA, and clinical professor of medicine and cardiology at the Medical College of Georgia. He is a fellow of the American College of Cardiology, American Heart Association, and the European Society of Cardiology, and a foundation fellow of the Ghana College of Physicians and Surgeons. Recent honours include the Distinguished Research Award of the International Society of Hypertension in Blacks, the 25th Bernard Pimstone Memorial Lecturer at the University of Cape Town in South Africa, and the National Heart Foundation of Australia Lecturer at the 50th Anniversary Celebration of the Cardiac Societies of Australia and New Zealand.

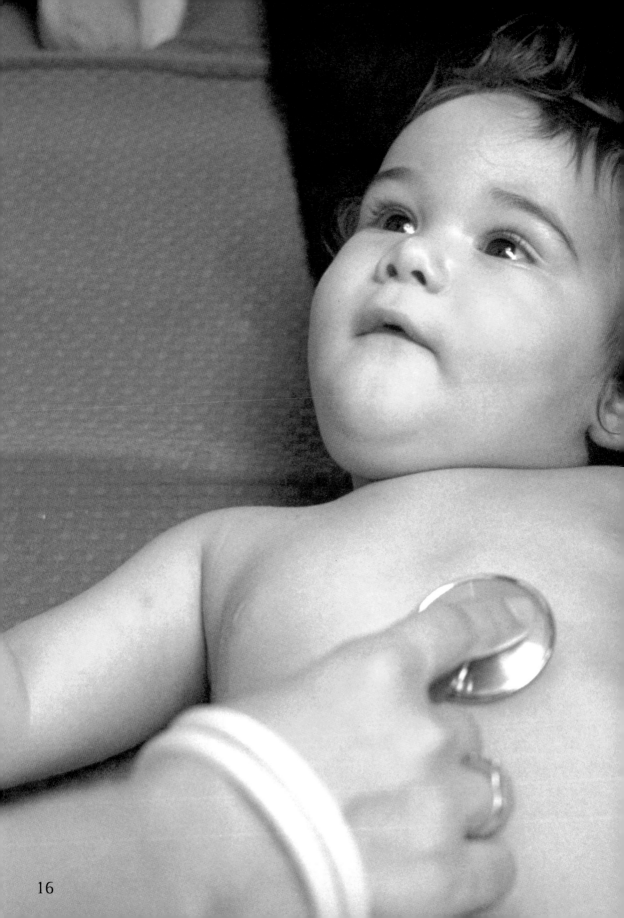

PART 1

CARDIOVASCULAR DISEASE

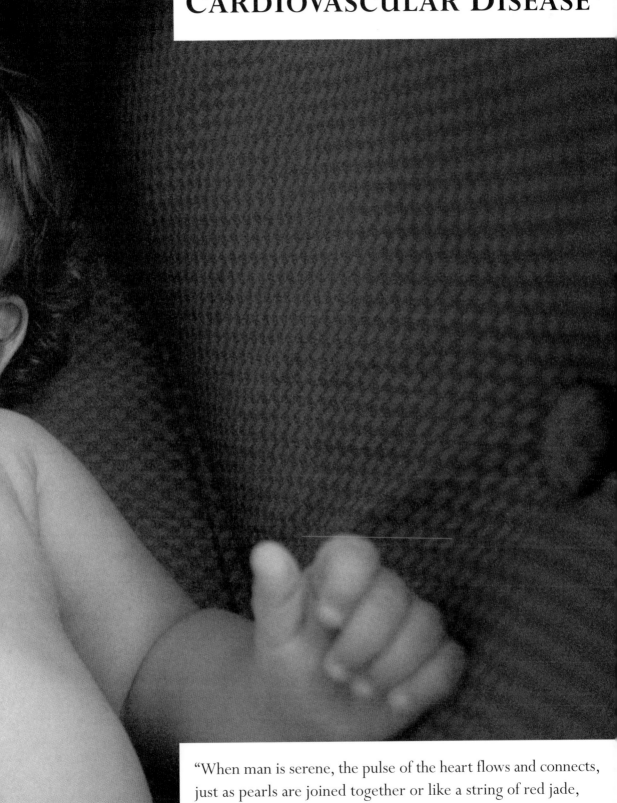

"When man is serene, the pulse of the heart flows and connects, just as pearls are joined together or like a string of red jade, then one can talk about a healthy heart."

The Yellow Emperor's *Canon of Internal Medicine*, 2500 BCE

1 Types of cardiovascular disease

The human heart is only the size of a fist, but it is the strongest muscle in the human body.

The heart starts to beat in the uterus long before birth, usually by 21 to 28 days after conception. The average heart beats about 100 000 times daily or about two and a half billion times over a 70 year lifetime.

With every heartbeat, the heart pumps blood around the body. It beats approximately 70 times a minute, although this rate can double during exercise or at times of extreme emotion.

Blood is pumped out from the left chambers of the heart. It is transported through arteries of ever-decreasing size, finally reaching the capillaries in all the tissues, such as the skin and other body organs. Having delivered its oxygen and nutrients and having collected waste products, blood is brought back to the right chambers of the heart through a system of ever-enlarging veins. During the circulation through the liver, waste products are removed.

This remarkable system is vulnerable to breakdown and assault from a variety of factors, many of which can be prevented and treated. Risk factors will be explored on pages 24–43.

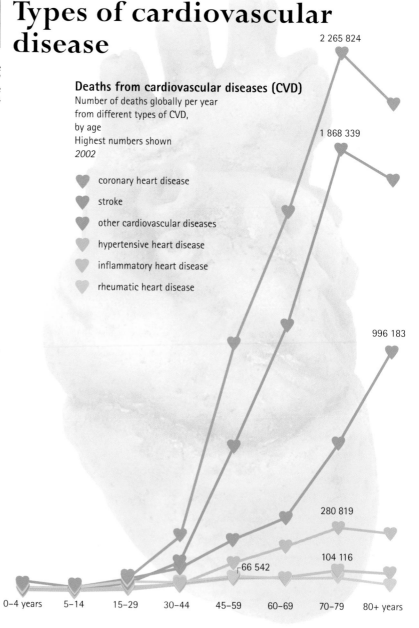

Deaths from cardiovascular diseases (CVD)
Number of deaths globally per year
from different types of CVD,
by age
Highest numbers shown
2002

- coronary heart disease
- stroke
- other cardiovascular diseases
- hypertensive heart disease
- inflammatory heart disease
- rheumatic heart disease

2 265 824
1 868 339
996 183
280 819
104 116
66 542

0–4 years | 5–14 | 15–29 | 30–44 | 45–59 | 60–69 | 70–79 | 80+ years

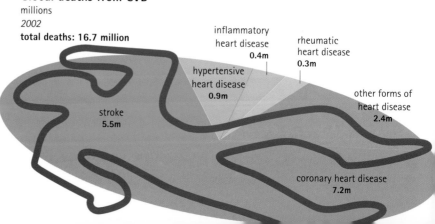

Global deaths from CVD
millions
2002
total deaths: 16.7 million

inflammatory heart disease 0.4m
rheumatic heart disease 0.3m
hypertensive heart disease 0.9m
other forms of heart disease 2.4m
stroke 5.5m
coronary heart disease 7.2m

Stroke

Strokes are caused by disruption of the blood supply to the brain. This may result from either blockage (ischaemic stroke) or rupture of a blood vessel (haemorrhagic stroke). *Risk factors* High blood pressure, atrial fibrillation (a heart rhythm disorder), high blood cholesterol, tobacco use, unhealthy diet, physical inactivity, diabetes, and advancing age.

Coronary heart disease kills more than 7 million people each year, and strokes kill nearly 6 million. Most of these deaths are in developing countries.

Coronary heart disease

Disease of the blood vessels supplying the heart muscle.
Major risk factors High blood pressure, high blood cholesterol, tobacco use, unhealthy diet, physical inactivity, diabetes, advancing age, inherited (genetic) disposition.
Other risk factors Poverty, low educational status, poor mental health (depression), inflammation and blood clotting disorders.

Rheumatic heart disease

Damage to the heart muscle and heart valves from rheumatic fever, caused by streptococcal bacteria.

Congenital heart disease

Malformations of heart structures existing at birth may be caused by genetic factors or by adverse exposures during gestation. Examples are holes in the heart, abnormal valves, and abnormal heart chambers.
Risk factors Maternal alcohol use, medicines (for example thalidomide, warfarin) used by the expectant mother, maternal infections such as rubella, poor maternal nutrition (low intake of folate), close blood relationship between parents (consanguinity).

Other cardiovascular diseases

Tumours of the heart; vascular tumours of the brain; disorders of heart muscle (cardiomyopathy); heart valve diseases; disorders of the lining of the heart.

Other factors that can damage the heart and blood vessel system

Inflammation, drugs, high blood pressure, unhealthy diet, trauma, toxins and alcohol.

Aortic aneurysm and dissection

Dilatation and rupture of the aorta.
Risk factors Advancing age, long-standing high blood pressure, Marfan syndrome, congenital heart disorders, syphilis, and other infectious and inflammatory disorders.

Peripheral arterial disease

Disease of the arteries supplying the arms and legs.
Risk factors As for coronary heart disease.

Deep venous thrombosis (DVT) and pulmonary embolism

Blood clots in the leg veins, which can dislodge and move to the heart and lungs.
Risk factors Surgery, obesity, cancer, previous episode of DVT, recent childbirth, use of oral contraceptive and hormone replacement therapy, long periods of immobility, for example while travelling, high homocysteine levels in the blood.

19

Rheumatic fever and rheumatic heart disease

Rheumatic fever usually follows an untreated beta-haemolytic streptococcal throat infection in children. It can affect many parts of the body, and may result in rheumatic heart disease, in which the heart valves are permanently damaged, and which may progress to heart failure, atrial fibrillation, and embolic stroke.

Nowadays, rheumatic fever mostly affects children in developing countries, especially where poverty is widespread. Up to 1% of all schoolchildren in Africa, Asia, the Eastern Mediterranean region and Latin America show signs of the disease.

Of 12 million people currently affected by rheumatic fever and rheumatic heart disease, two-thirds are children between 5 and 15 years of age. There are around 300 000 deaths each year, with two million people requiring repeated hospitalization and one million likely to require surgery in the next 5 to 20 years.

Early treatment of streptococcal sore throat can preclude the development of rheumatic fever. Regular long-term penicillin treatment can prevent rheumatic fever becoming rheumatic heart disease, and can halt disease progression in people whose heart valves are already damaged by the disease. In many developing countries, lack of awareness of these measures, coupled with shortages of money and resources, are important barriers to the control of the disease.

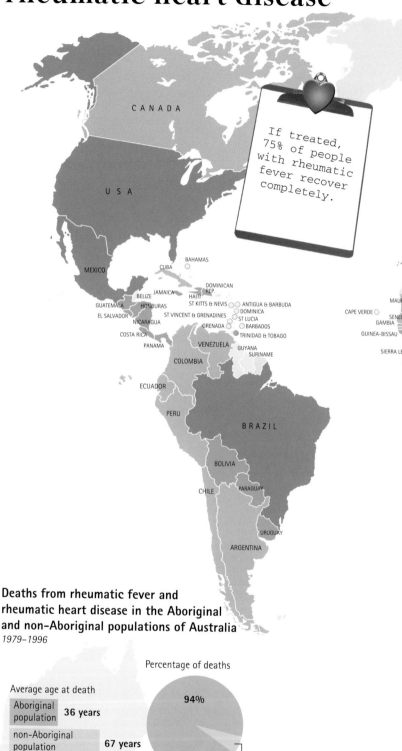

If treated, 75% of people with rheumatic fever recover completely.

Deaths from rheumatic fever and rheumatic heart disease in the Aboriginal and non-Aboriginal populations of Australia
1979–1996

Average age at death

| Aboriginal population | 36 years |
| non-Aboriginal population | 67 years |

Percentage of deaths

94%

6%

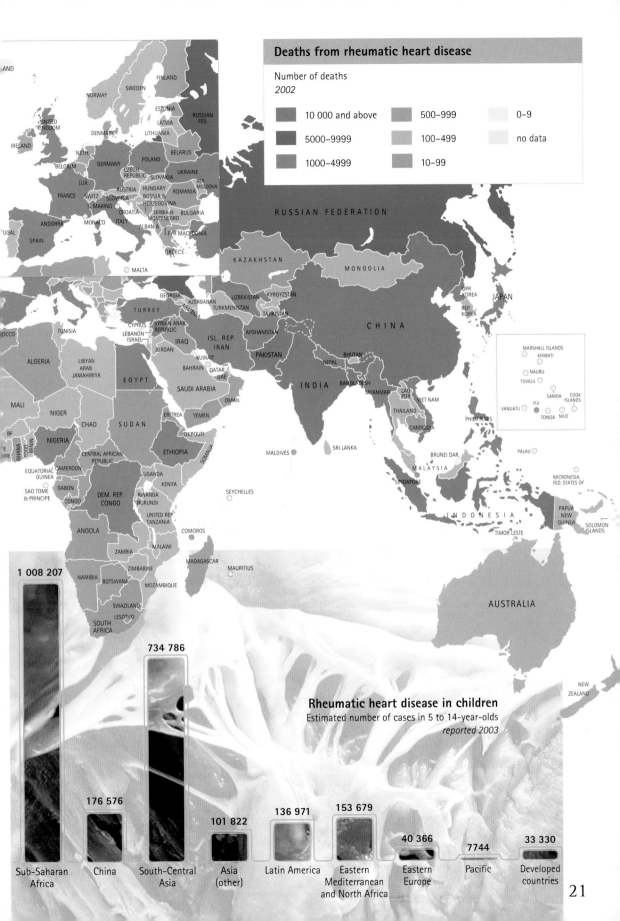

Deaths from rheumatic heart disease

Number of deaths
2002

10 000 and above	
5000–9999	
1000–4999	
500–999	
100–499	
10–99	
0–9	
no data	

Rheumatic heart disease in children
Estimated number of cases in 5 to 14-year-olds
reported 2003

1 008 207 — Sub-Saharan Africa
176 576 — China
734 786 — South-Central Asia
101 822 — Asia (other)
136 971 — Latin America
153 679 — Eastern Mediterranean and North Africa
40 366 — Eastern Europe
7744 — Pacific
33 330 — Developed countries

21

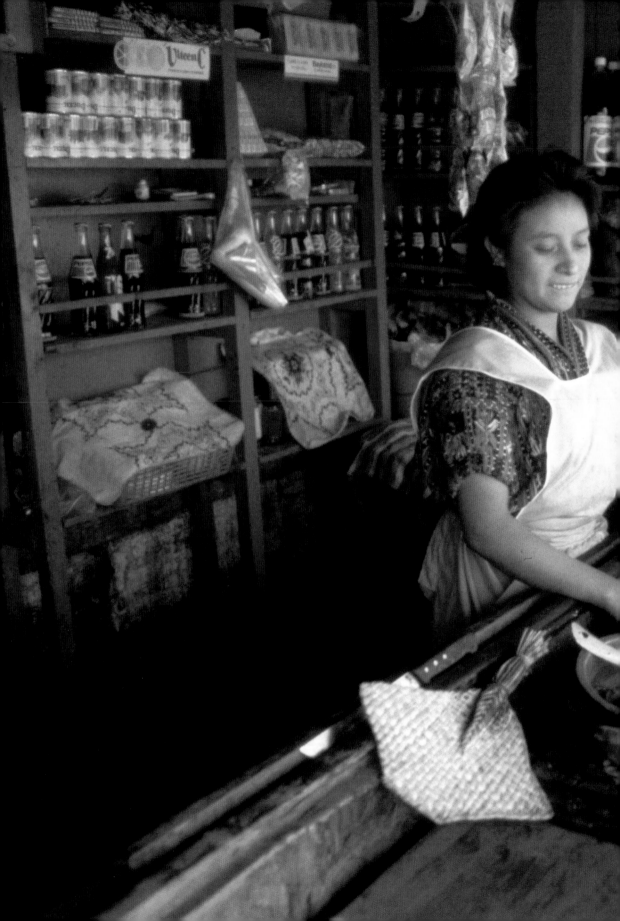

PART 2

RISK FACTORS

"He that eats but one dish seldom needs the doctor."
Old Scottish proverb

Risk factors

Over 300 risk factors have been associated with coronary heart disease and stroke. The major established risk factors meet three criteria: a high prevalence in many populations; a significant independent impact on the risk of coronary heart disease or stroke; and their treatment and control result in reduced risk.

Risk factors for cardiovascular disease are now significant in all populations. In the developed countries, at least one-third of all CVD is attributable to five risk factors: tobacco use, alcohol use, high blood pressure, high cholesterol and obesity.

In developing countries with low mortality, such as China, cardiovascular risk factors also figure high on the top 10 list. These populations face a double burden of risks, grappling with the problems of undernutrition and communicable diseases, while also contending with the same risks as developed nations.

Even in developing countries with high mortality, such as those in sub-Saharan Africa, high blood pressure, high cholesterol, tobacco and alcohol use, as well as low vegetable and fruit intake, already figure among the top risk factors.

Some major risks are modifiable in that they can be prevented, treated, and controlled. There are considerable health benefits at all ages, for both men and women, in stopping smoking, reducing cholesterol and blood pressure, eating a healthy diet and increasing physical activity.

Leading risk factors
As percentage burden of all diseases
2002

major CVD risk factors
other risk factors

2.5% high blood pressure
2.0% tobacco use
1.9% high cholesterol
14.9% underweight
10.2% unsafe sex
5.5% unsafe water, sanitation & hygiene
3.7% indoor smoke from solid fuels
3.2% zinc deficiency
3.1% iron deficiency
3.0% vitamin A deficiency

High-mortality developing countries

5.0% high blood pressure
4.0% tobacco use
2.1% high cholesterol
6.2% alcohol
2.7% obesity
1.9% low fruit & vegetable intake
3.1% underweight
1.9% indoor smoke from solid fuels
1.8% iron deficiency
1.7% unsafe water, sanitation & hygiene

Low-mortality developing countries

10.9% high blood pressure
12.2% tobacco use
7.6% high cholesterol
9.2% alcohol
7.4% obesity
3.9% low fruit & vegetable intake
3.3% physical inactivity
1.8% illicit drug use
0.8% unsafe sex
0.7% iron deficiency

Developed countries

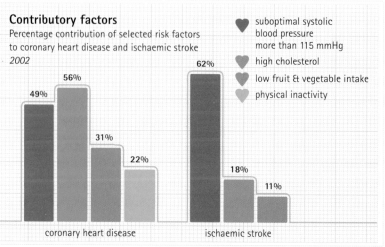

Contributory factors
Percentage contribution of selected risk factors to coronary heart disease and ischaemic stroke
2002

suboptimal systolic blood pressure more than 115 mmHg
high cholesterol
low fruit & vegetable intake
physical inactivity

49% 56% 31% 22% — coronary heart disease
62% 18% 11% — ischaemic stroke

Major modifiable risk factors

- **High blood pressure**
  Major risk for heart attack and the most important risk factor for stroke.
- **Abnormal blood lipids**
  High total cholesterol, LDL-cholesterol and triglyceride levels, and low levels of HDL-cholesterol increase risk of coronary heart disease and ischaemic stroke.
- **Tobacco use**
  Increases risks of cardiovascular disease, especially in people who started young, and heavy smokers. Passive smoking an additional risk.
- **Physical inactivity**
  Increases risk of heart disease and stroke by 50%.

- **Obesity**
  Major risk for coronary heart disease and diabetes.
- **Unhealthy diets**
  Low fruit and vegetable intake is estimated to cause about 31% of coronary heart disease and 11% of stroke worldwide; high saturated fat intake increases the risk of heart disease and stroke through its effect on blood lipids and thrombosis.
- **Diabetes mellitus**
  Major risk for coronary heart disease and stroke.

Approximately 75% of cardiovascular disease can be attributed to conventional risk factors.

Other modifiable risk factors

- **Low socioeconomic status (SES)**
  Consistent inverse relationship with risk of heart disease and stroke.
- **Mental ill-health**
  Depression is associated with an increased risk of coronary heart disease.
- **Psychosocial stress**
  Chronic life stress, social isolation and anxiety increase the risk of heart disease and stroke.

- **Alcohol use**
  One to two drinks per day may lead to a 30% reduction in heart disease, but heavy drinking damages the heart muscle.
- **Use of certain medication**
  Some oral contraceptives and hormone replacement therapy increase risk of heart disease.
- **Lipoprotein(a)**
  Increases risk of heart attacks especially in presence of high LDL-cholesterol.
- **Left ventricular hypertrophy (LVH)**
  A powerful marker of cardiovascular death.

Non-modifiable risk factors

- **Advancing age**
  Most powerful independent risk factor for cardiovascular disease; risk of stroke doubles every decade after age 55.
- **Heredity or family history**
  Increased risk if a first-degree blood relative has had coronary heart disease or stroke before the age of 55 years (for a male relative) or 65 years (for a female relative).

- **Gender**
  Higher rates of coronary heart disease among men compared with women (premenopausal age); risk of stroke is similar for men and women.
- **Ethnicity or race**
  Increased stroke noted for Blacks, some Hispanic Americans, Chinese, and Japanese populations. Increased cardiovascular disease deaths noted for South Asians and American Blacks in comparison with Whites.

"Novel" risk factors

- **Excess homocysteine in blood**
  High levels may be associated with an increase in cardiovascular risk.
- **Inflammation**
  Several inflammatory markers are associated with increased cardiovascular risk, e.g. elevated C-reactive protein (CRP).

- **Abnormal blood coagulation**
  Elevated blood levels of fibrinogen and other markers of blood clotting increase the risk of cardiovascular complications.

Risk factors start in childhood and youth

Although cardiovascular diseases typically occur in middle age or later, risk factors are determined to a great extent by behaviours learned in childhood and continued into adulthood, such as dietary habits and smoking.

Throughout the world, these risks are starting to appear earlier. Physical activity decreases markedly in adolescence, particularly in girls. Obesity has increased substantially, not only in Europe and North America, but also in traditionally slender populations such as the Chinese and Japanese. Type 2 diabetes was previously rare in children, but is increasing in adolescents in, for example, North America, Japan and Thailand.

Markers of CVD can be seen in young children. Post-mortems of children who died in accidents have found fatty streaks and fibrous plaques in the coronary arteries. These early lesions of atherosclerosis were most frequently found in children whose risk factors included smoking, elevated plasma lipids, high blood pressure and obesity.

Programmes to address childhood and youth risk factors are mostly confined to developed countries, but urgent action is required worldwide. Families, schools, communities, health professionals, public health officials and policy-makers all need to promote healthy lifestyles in children and young people. Unless the spread of risk factors is stemmed, the world faces an epidemic of CVD.

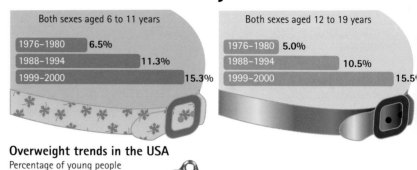

Both sexes aged 6 to 11 years		Both sexes aged 12 to 19 years	
1976–1980	6.5%	1976–1980	5.0%
1988–1994	11.3%	1988–1994	10.5%
1999–2000	15.3%	1999–2000	15.5%

Overweight trends in the USA
Percentage of young people who are overweight
1976–2000

The risks for cardiovascular disease start in youth: worldwide, 18 million children under five years old are overweight, and 14% of 13 to 15-year-old students around the world currently smoke cigarettes.

Overweight youth
Percentage of 15-year-olds who are overweight
1997–1998
selected countries

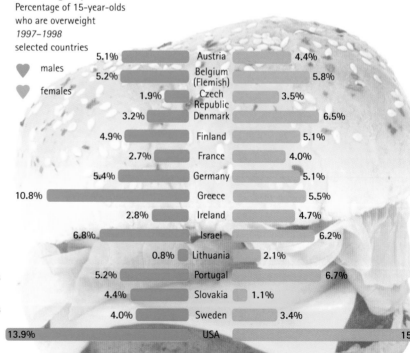

♥ males
♥ females

	males	Country	females
	5.1%	Austria	4.4%
	5.2%	Belgium (Flemish)	5.8%
	1.9%	Czech Republic	3.5%
	3.2%	Denmark	6.5%
	4.9%	Finland	5.1%
	2.7%	France	4.0%
	5.4%	Germany	5.1%
10.8%		Greece	5.5%
	2.8%	Ireland	4.7%
	6.8%	Israel	6.2%
	0.8%	Lithuania	2.1%
	5.2%	Portugal	6.7%
	4.4%	Slovakia	1.1%
	4.0%	Sweden	3.4%
13.9%		USA	15.1%

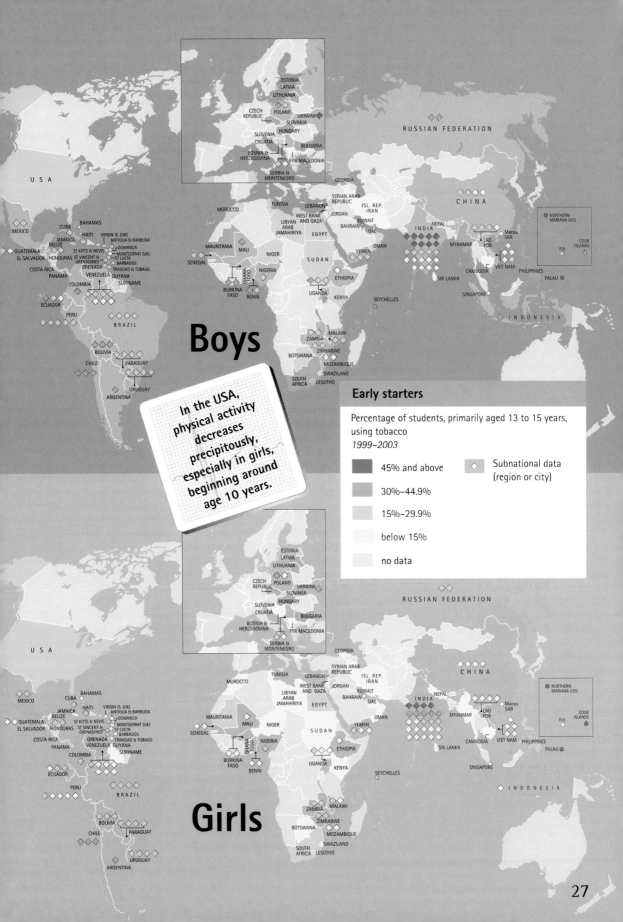

Boys

Girls

In the USA, physical activity decreases precipitously, especially in girls, beginning around age 10 years.

Early starters

Percentage of students, primarily aged 13 to 15 years, using tobacco
1999–2003

- 45% and above
- 30%–44.9%
- 15%–29.9%
- below 15%
- no data

◇ Subnational data (region or city)

Risk factor: blood pressure

High blood pressure (hypertension) is one of the most important preventable causes of premature death worldwide. Even a blood pressure at the top end of the normal range increases risk. High blood pressure is defined as a systolic blood pressure (SBP) above 140 mmHg and/or a diastolic blood pressure (DBP) above 90 mmHg.

In most countries, up to 30% of adults suffer from high blood pressure and a further 50% to 60% would be in better health if they reduced their blood pressure, by increasing physical activity, maintaining an ideal body weight and eating more fruits and vegetables.

In people aged up to 50 years, both DBP and SBP are associated with cardiovascular risk; above this age, SBP is a far more important predictor. Blood pressure usually rises with age, except where salt intake is low, physical activity high, and obesity largely absent.

Most natural foods contain salt, but processed food may be high in salt; in addition, individuals may add salt for taste. Dietary salt increases blood pressure in most people with hypertension, and in about a quarter of those with normal blood pressure, especially with increasing age. A high intake of salt independently increases the risk of CVD in overweight persons.

In addition to lifestyle changes, effective medication is available for control of high blood pressure.

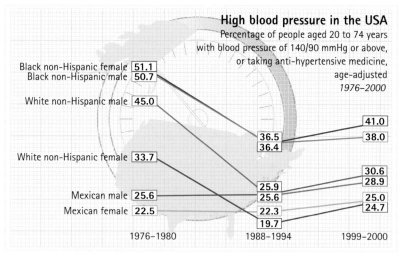

High blood pressure in the USA
Percentage of people aged 20 to 74 years with blood pressure of 140/90 mmHg or above, or taking anti-hypertensive medicine, age-adjusted
1976–2000

	1976–1980	1988–1994	1999–2000
Black non-Hispanic female	51.1		
Black non-Hispanic male	50.7		41.0
White non-Hispanic male	45.0	36.5	38.0
		36.4	
White non-Hispanic female	33.7		30.6
		25.9	28.9
Mexican male	25.6	25.6	25.0
Mexican female	22.5	22.3	24.7
		19.7	

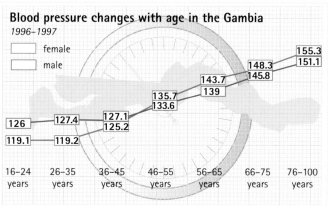

Blood pressure changes with age in the Gambia
1996–1997

☐ female
☐ male

16–24 years	26–35 years	36–45 years	46–55 years	56–65 years	66–75 years	76–100 years
126	127.4	127.1	135.7	143.7	148.3	155.3
119.1	119.2	125.2	133.6	139	145.8	151.1

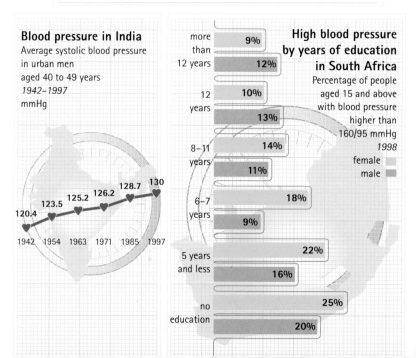

Blood pressure in India
Average systolic blood pressure in urban men aged 40 to 49 years
1942–1997
mmHg

1942	1954	1963	1971	1985	1997
120.4	123.5	125.2	126.2	128.7	130

High blood pressure by years of education in South Africa
Percentage of people aged 15 and above with blood pressure higher than 160/95 mmHg
1998

female ▭
male ▭

	female	male
more than 12 years	9%	12%
12 years	10%	13%
8–11 years	14%	11%
6–7 years	18%	9%
5 years and less	22%	16%
no education	25%	20%

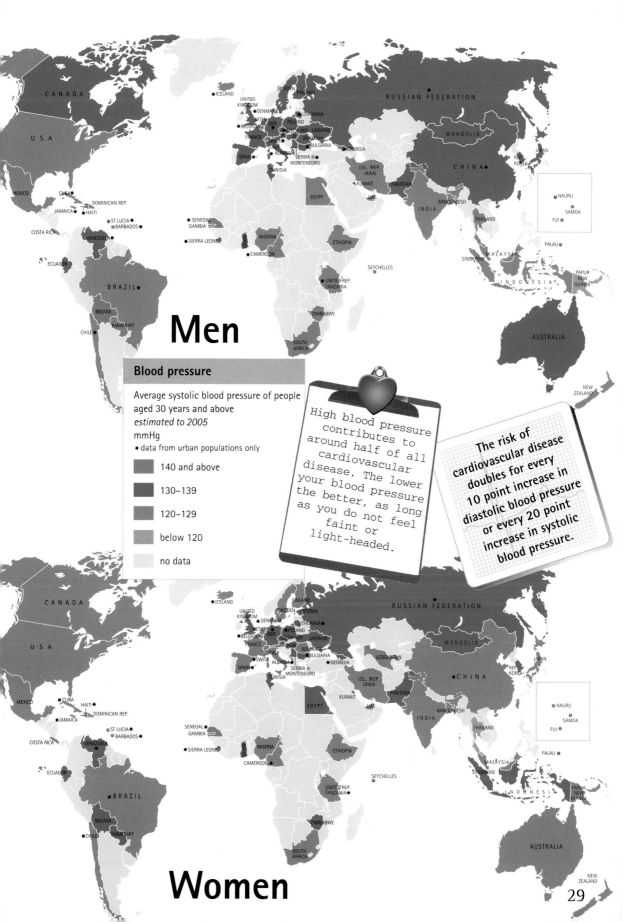

Men

Blood pressure

Average systolic blood pressure of people aged 30 years and above
estimated to 2005
mmHg
✱ data from urban populations only

- 140 and above
- 130–139
- 120–129
- below 120
- no data

High blood pressure contributes to around half of all cardiovascular disease. The lower your blood pressure the better, as long as you do not feel faint or light-headed.

The risk of cardiovascular disease doubles for every 10 point increase in diastolic blood pressure or every 20 point increase in systolic blood pressure.

Women

Risk factor: lipids

High levels of LDL-cholesterol, and other abnormal lipids (fats), are risk factors for cardiovascular disease. Cholesterol is a soft, waxy substance found among the lipids in the bloodstream and in all the body's cells. It is needed to form cell membranes and hormones, and for other bodily functions.

The body can make cholesterol, or it can obtain it from food, especially animal products such as meats, poultry, fish, eggs, and dairy products. Certain saturated vegetable fats and oils, including coconut fat and palm oil, are cholesterol-free but cause an increase in blood cholesterol. Some foods that do not contain animal products may contain trans-fats, which also cause the body to make more cholesterol. Fruit, vegetables and cereals do not contain cholesterol.

Cholesterol is transported around the body in two kinds of lipoproteins: low-density lipoprotein, or LDL, and high-density lipoprotein, or HDL. A high level of LDL can lead to clogging of the arteries, increasing the risk of heart attack and ischaemic stroke, while HDL reduces the risk of coronary heart disease and stroke.

The female sex hormone estrogen tends to raise HDL-cholesterol levels, which may help explain why premenopausal women are relatively protected from developing coronary heart disease.

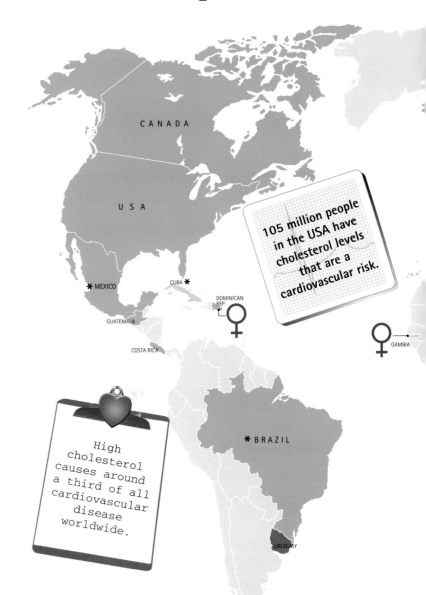

105 million people in the USA have cholesterol levels that are a cardiovascular risk.

High cholesterol causes around a third of all cardiovascular disease worldwide.

Current recommended lipid levels

	European guideline	US guideline
Total cholesterol	less than 5.0 mmol/l	less than 240 mg/dl (6.2 mmol/l)
LDL-cholesterol	less than 3.0 mmol/l	less than 160 mg/dl (3.8 mmol/l)
HDL-cholesterol	1.0 mmol/l or more in males 1.2 mmol/l or more in females	40 mg/dl (1 mmol/l) or more
Triglycerides (fasting)	less than 1.7 mmol/l	less than 200 mg/dl (2.3 mmol/l)

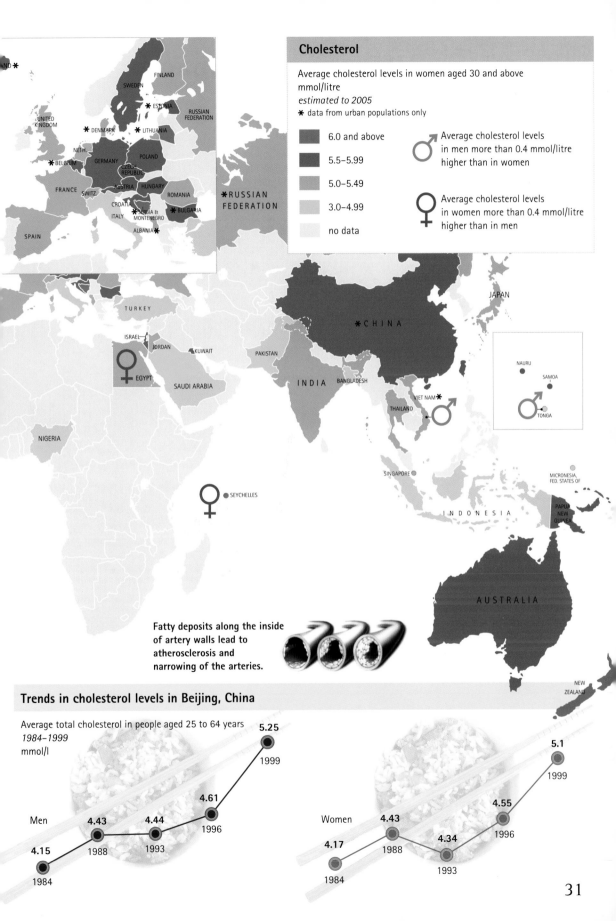

Cholesterol

Average cholesterol levels in women aged 30 and above
mmol/litre
estimated to 2005
✳ data from urban populations only

■	6.0 and above
■	5.5–5.99
■	5.0–5.49
■	3.0–4.99
■	no data

♂ Average cholesterol levels
in men more than 0.4 mmol/litre
higher than in women

♀ Average cholesterol levels
in women more than 0.4 mmol/litre
higher than in men

Fatty deposits along the inside
of artery walls lead to
atherosclerosis and
narrowing of the arteries.

Trends in cholesterol levels in Beijing, China

Average total cholesterol in people aged 25 to 64 years
1984–1999
mmol/l

Men
4.15 1984
4.43 1988
4.44 1993
4.61 1996
5.25 1999

Women
4.17 1984
4.43 1988
4.34 1993
4.55 1996
5.1 1999

Risk factor: tobacco

The public may believe that the major risk from cigarettes is lung cancer, but far more smokers develop cardiovascular disease – mainly heart attacks and stroke. In 1940, a link was identified between cigarette use and coronary heart disease, and there is now a huge body of scientific literature linking tobacco with CVD. The risks are much higher in people who started smoking before the age of 16. Tobacco use, other than smoking, and passive smoking are also implicated as CVD risks.

Smoking promotes CVD through several mechanisms. It damages the endothelium lining of the blood vessels, increases cholesterol plaques (fatty deposits in the arteries), increases clotting, raises LDL-cholesterol levels and lowers HDL, and promotes coronary artery spasm. Nicotine accelerates the heart rate and raises blood pressure.

A gene has been discovered that increases smokers' risk of developing coronary heart disease by up to four times. Around a quarter of the population carries one or more copies of this gene.

Women smokers are at particular risk, with a higher risk of heart attack than male smokers. Women who smoke only three to five cigarettes a day double their risk of heart attack, while men who smoke six to nine cigarettes a day double their risk.

Cardiovascular risks of smoking

Percentage increase in risk

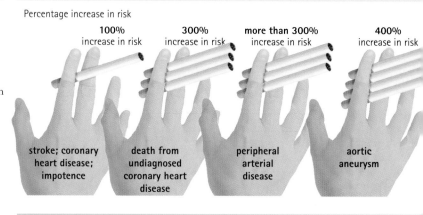

100% increase in risk	300% increase in risk	more than 300% increase in risk	400% increase in risk
stroke; coronary heart disease; impotence	death from undiagnosed coronary heart disease	peripheral arterial disease	aortic aneurysm

Cardiovascular risks of passive smoking

Adults
- Harms, clogs, and weakens arteries
- Heart attack, angina, stroke

Children
- Reduces amount of oxygen the blood can carry
- Damages arteries
- Early-onset atherosclerosis
- Sudden infant death syndrome (cot death)

In the USA, up to 62 000 people die each year from heart disease caused by passive smoking.

Smokers don't know the risks of heart attack

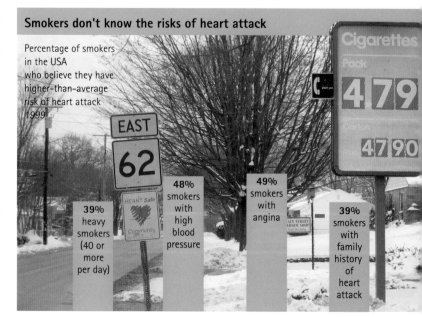

Percentage of smokers in the USA who believe they have higher-than-average risk of heart attack 1999

- 39% heavy smokers (40 or more per day)
- 48% smokers with high blood pressure
- 49% smokers with angina
- 39% smokers with family history of heart attack

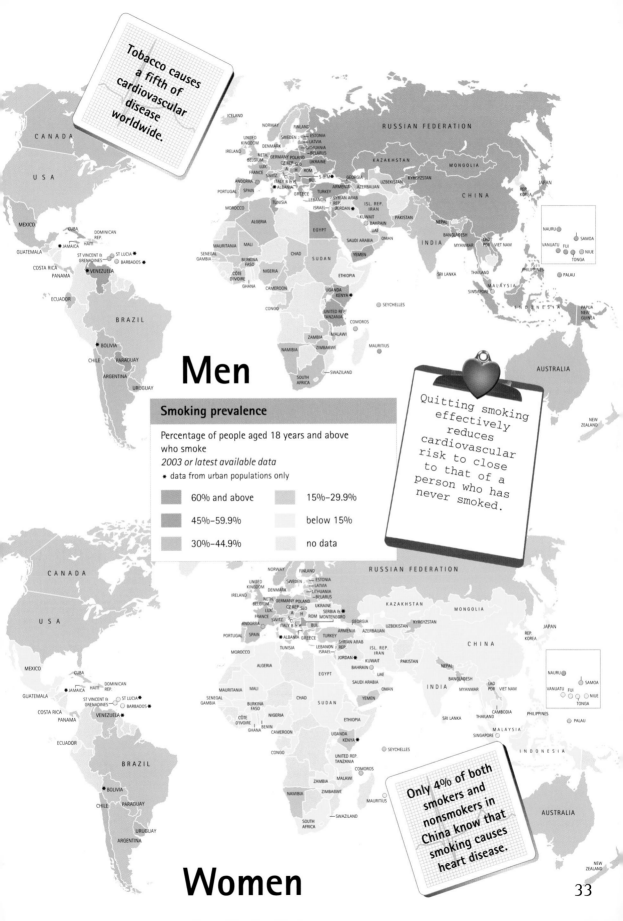

Tobacco causes a fifth of cardiovascular disease worldwide.

Men

Smoking prevalence

Percentage of people aged 18 years and above who smoke
2003 or latest available data
* data from urban populations only

- 60% and above
- 45%–59.9%
- 30%–44.9%
- 15%–29.9%
- below 15%
- no data

Quitting smoking effectively reduces cardiovascular risk to close to that of a person who has never smoked.

Only 4% of both smokers and nonsmokers in China know that smoking causes heart disease.

Women

33

Risk factor: physical inactivity

Industrialization, urbanization and mechanized transport have reduced physical activity, even in developing countries, so that currently more than 60% of the global population are not sufficiently active.

Physical exercise is linked to longevity, independently of genetic factors. Physical activity, even at an older age, can significantly reduce the risk of coronary heart disease, diabetes, high blood pressure, and obesity, help reduce stress, anxiety and depression, and improve lipid profile. It also reduces the risks of colon cancer, breast cancer and ischaemic stroke.

Doing more than 150 minutes of moderate physical activity or 60 minutes of vigorous physical activity a week – whether at work, in the home, or elsewhere – can reduce the risk of coronary heart disease by approximately 30%.

Despite documented evidence of the benefit of physical activity in preventing and treating cardiovascular and other chronic diseases, more than a quarter of a million individuals die each year in the United States because of a "lack of regular physical exercise".

Only 8% of the world's population currently owns a car. Between 1980 and 1998, the global fleet of cars, trucks and buses grew by 80%, with a third of the increase taking place in developing countries.

Sitting

Time spent seated each week, people aged 18 years and above
2000
selected countries

31 hours	29 hours	37 hours	42 hours	35 hours
Finland, France	Italy	Netherlands	Spain	United Kingdom

Physical activity

The following activities have similar benefits to health:

Washing and waxing a car for 45–60 minutes

Washing windows or floors for 45–60 minutes

Playing volleyball for 45 minutes

Wheeling self in wheelchair for 30–40 minutes

Bicycling 8 km in 30 minutes

Pushing a pushchair 2.5 km in 30 minutes

Walking 3 km in 30 minutes

Swimming laps for 20 minutes

Playing basketball for 15–20 minutes

Physical inactivity by social class in India

Percentage of time spent seated, at work or in spare time, by people aged 25 years and above in two Indian villages
1993–1995

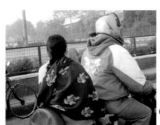

♥ male
♡ female

4% 3%	6% 6%	27% 69%	37% 82%
lowest	next lowest	next highest	highest

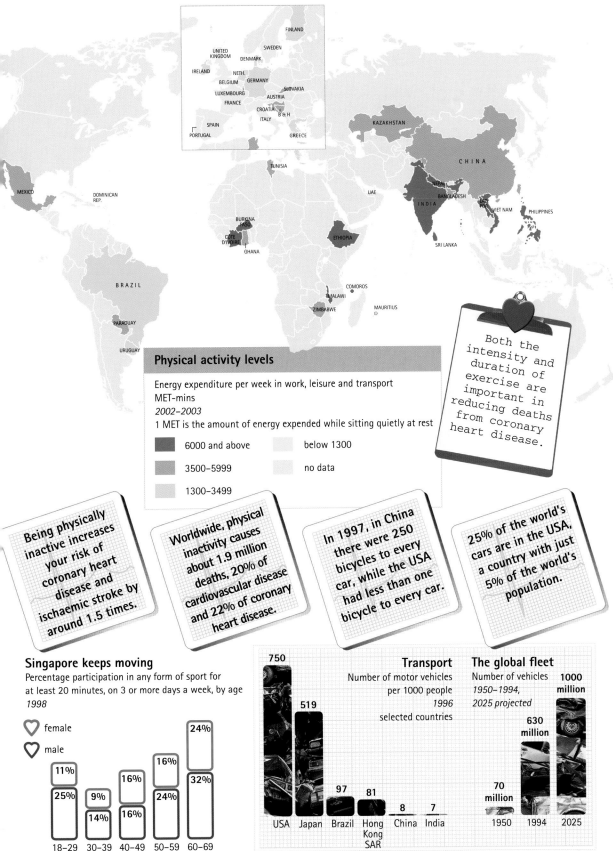

Physical activity levels

Energy expenditure per week in work, leisure and transport
MET-mins
2002–2003
1 MET is the amount of energy expended while sitting quietly at rest

6000 and above		below 1300
3500–5999		no data
1300–3499		

Both the intensity and duration of exercise are important in reducing deaths from coronary heart disease.

Being physically inactive increases your risk of coronary heart disease and ischaemic stroke by around 1.5 times.

Worldwide, physical inactivity causes about 1.9 million deaths, 20% of cardiovascular disease and 22% of coronary heart disease.

In 1997, in China there were 250 bicycles to every car, while the USA had less than one bicycle to every car.

25% of the world's cars are in the USA, a country with just 5% of the world's population.

Singapore keeps moving

Percentage participation in any form of sport for at least 20 minutes, on 3 or more days a week, by age
1998

♥ female
♥ male

				24%
11%		16%	16%	
25%	9%	16%	24%	32%
	14%	16%		
18–29 years	30–39 years	40–49 years	50–59 years	60–69 years

Transport
Number of motor vehicles per 1000 people
1996
selected countries

USA	Japan	Brazil	Hong Kong SAR	China	India
750	519	97	81	8	7

The global fleet
Number of vehicles
*1950–1994,
2025 projected*

1950	1994	2025
70 million	630 million	1000 million

Risk factor: obesity

"Eat less at dinner and you will live to ninety-nine."
Ancient Chinese proverb

Belt size, abdominal girth and waist-to-hip ratio are useful indicators of obesity. The Body Mass Index (BMI), a measure of weight in relation to height, is commonly used for classifying overweight and obesity.

The risks of cardiovascular disease and type 2 diabetes tend to increase on a continuum with increasing BMI, but for practical purposes a person with a BMI of over 25 is considered overweight, while someone with a BMI of over 30 is obese. But one size does not fit all. In women, a BMI as low as 21 may be associated with the greatest protection from coronary heart disease death. The BMI for observed risk in different Asian populations varies from 22 to 25 kg/m².

Availability of food, changes in the kind of food eaten, and decreased exercise are presenting humanity with one of its greatest challenges. Low fruit and vegetable intake accounts for about 20% of CVD worldwide. Obese smokers live 14 fewer years than nonsmokers of normal weight.

More than 60% of adults in the USA are overweight or obese. Triple-width coffins, capable of holding a 300 kg (700 lb) body, are in increasing demand. Worldwide, airlines are having to recalculate their passenger "payload" weight. There are 70 million overweight people in China. South Pacific populations used to be physically active and slim, but the region now has some of the world's highest rates of obesity.

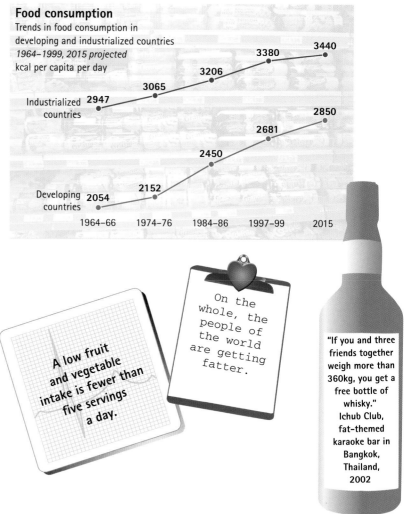

Food consumption

Trends in food consumption in developing and industrialized countries
1964–1999, 2015 projected
kcal per capita per day

Industrialized countries: 2947, 3065, 3206, 3380, 3440

Developing countries: 2054, 2152, 2450, 2681, 2850

1964–66 1974–76 1984–86 1997–99 2015

A low fruit and vegetable intake is fewer than five servings a day.

On the whole, the people of the world are getting fatter.

"If you and three friends together weigh more than 360kg, you get a free bottle of whisky."
Ichub Club, fat-themed karaoke bar in Bangkok, Thailand, 2002

Apple shape at higher risk of CVD than pear shape

Waist-to-hip ratio of 0.91 and above is associated with nearly threefold increased risk of coronary heart disease.

Increased CVD risk if:	Men	Women
Waist to hip ratio	more than 0.90	more than 0.85
Waist measurement	more than 101cm (40 inches)	more than 89cm (35 inches)

Cartoon characters used to promote the WeightWise campaign of the British Dietetic Association.

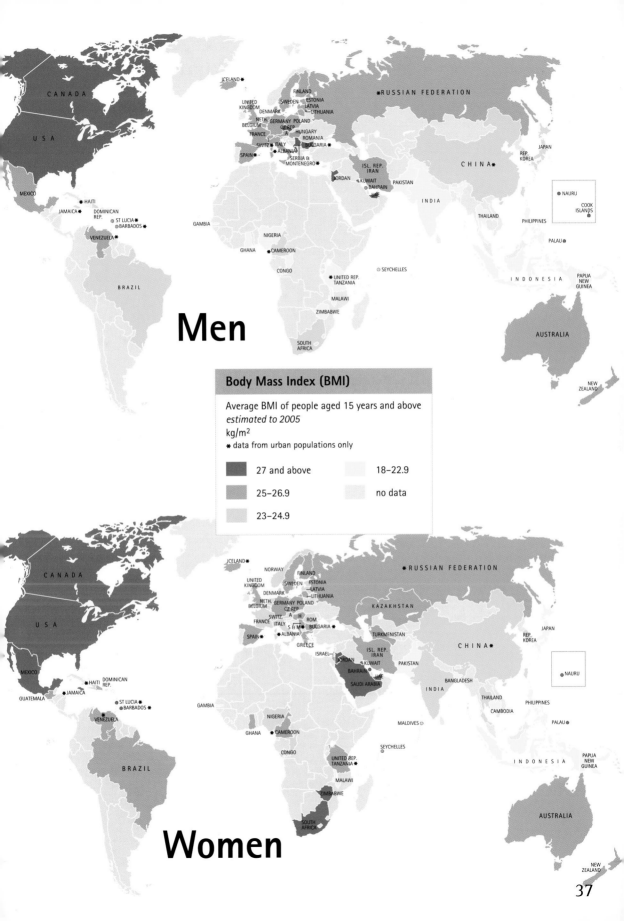

Men

Body Mass Index (BMI)

Average BMI of people aged 15 years and above
estimated to 2005
kg/m²

✳ data from urban populations only

■ 27 and above		■ 18–22.9
■ 25–26.9		■ no data
■ 23–24.9		

Women

37

"The urine of diabetics is wonderfully sweet as if imbued with honey or sugar."
Thomas Willis (1621–1675), physician to King Charles II, England

Diabetes is a risk factor for coronary heart disease and stroke, and is the most common cause of amputation that is not the result of an accident.

Insulin is a hormone produced by the pancreas and used by the body to regulate glucose (sugar). Diabetes occurs when the body does not produce enough insulin, or cannot use it properly, leading to too much sugar in the blood. Symptoms include thirst, excessive urination, tiredness, and unexplained weight loss.

There are two main types of diabetes. Type 1 diabetes, in which the pancreas stops making insulin, accounts for 10% to 15% of cases. The majority of people with diabetes have type 2 disease, in which insulin is produced in smaller amounts than needed, or is not properly effective. This form is preventable, because it is related to physical inactivity, excess calorie intake and obesity. People with type 1 diabetes need insulin injections to lower blood sugar, but many people with type 2 do not.

At least half of all people with diabetes are unaware of their condition. Diabetes is more prevalent in developed countries, but modernization and lifestyle changes are likely to result in a future epidemic of diabetes in developing countries.

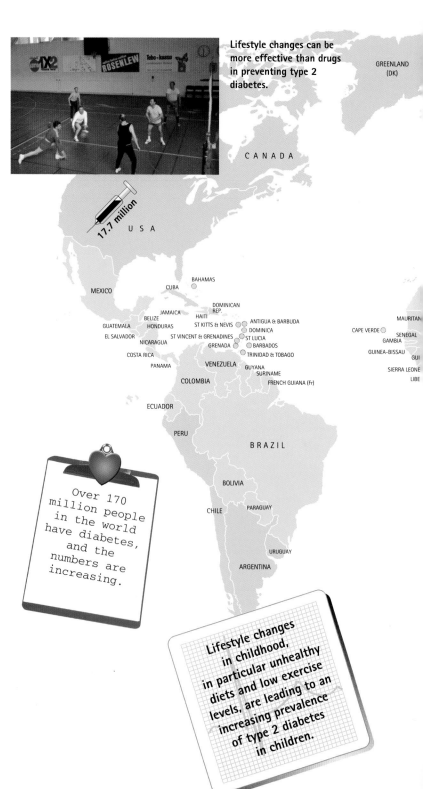

Lifestyle changes can be more effective than drugs in preventing type 2 diabetes.

17.7 million — USA

Over 170 million people in the world have diabetes, and the numbers are increasing.

Lifestyle changes in childhood, in particular unhealthy diets and low exercise levels, are leading to an increasing prevalence of type 2 diabetes in children.

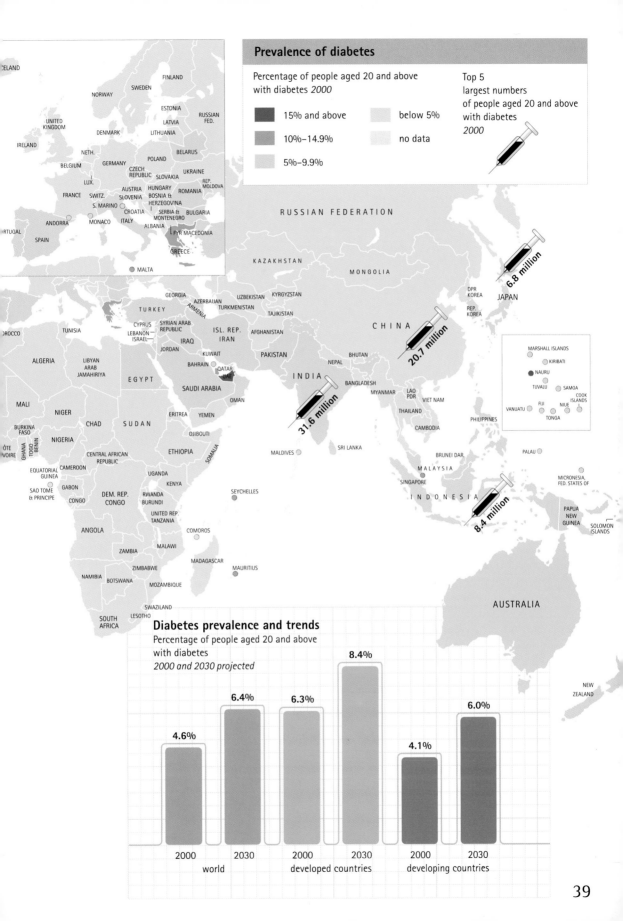

Prevalence of diabetes

Percentage of people aged 20 and above
with diabetes *2000*

- 15% and above
- 10%–14.9%
- 5%–9.9%
- below 5%
- no data

Top 5
largest numbers
of people aged 20 and above
with diabetes
2000

6.8 million (JAPAN)

20.7 million (CHINA)

31.6 million (INDIA)

8.4 million (INDONESIA)

Diabetes prevalence and trends

Percentage of people aged 20 and above
with diabetes
2000 and 2030 projected

	world		developed countries		developing countries
2000	2030	2000	2030	2000	2030
4.6%	6.4%	6.3%	8.4%	4.1%	6.0%

Risk factor: socioeconomic status

"Wealth is both an enemy and a friend."
Nepalese proverb

In developing countries, coronary heart disease has historically been more common in the more educated and higher socioeconomic groups, but this is beginning to change. In industrial countries, such as Canada, the United Kingdom, and the United States, there is a widening social class difference in the opposite direction.

Studies in developed countries suggest that low income is associated with a higher incidence of coronary heart disease, and with higher mortality after a heart attack. The prevalence of risk factors for heart disease, such as high blood pressure, smoking and diabetes, is also higher. The use of medications is lower, especially of lipid-lowering agents and ACE inhibitors, as well as other treatments, such as cardiac catheterization.

The pathways by which socioeconomic status might affect cardiovascular disease include: lifestyle and behaviour patterns; ease of access to health care; and chronic stress.

In Canada, children from poor families are twice as likely to be obese as children from rich families.

Low socioeconomic status is associated with increased risk of cardiovascular disease.

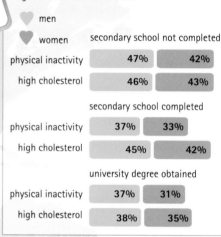

Prevalence of CVD risk factors by education in Canada

Percentage of people aged 18 to 74 years with high levels of physical inactivity and high cholesterol, by educational level, age standardized *1986–1992*

♥ men
♥ women

secondary school not completed

	men	women
physical inactivity	47%	42%
high cholesterol	46%	43%

secondary school completed

	men	women
physical inactivity	37%	33%
high cholesterol	45%	42%

university degree obtained

	men	women
physical inactivity	37%	31%
high cholesterol	38%	35%

The CVD mortality gap in the USA

Percentage increased CVD mortality of lowest socioeconomic (SE) group over highest SE group, in people aged 25 to 64 years *1969–1998*

♥ women
♥ men

	1969–1970	1997–1998
women	49%	94%
men	30%	79%

Prevalence of high blood pressure by income in Trinidad and Tobago

Percentage of women aged 24 to 85 years with blood pressure of 140/90 mmHg or above, or currently treated
2001

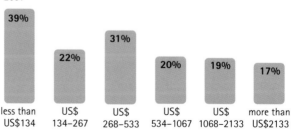

monthly household income					
less than US$134	US$ 134–267	US$ 268–533	US$ 534–1067	US$ 1068–2133	more than US$2133
39%	22%	31%	20%	19%	17%

Educational level and obesity in Italy

Percentage increased risk of obesity in people aged 35 to 74 years, in comparison with university graduates
1998

💗 women
💗 men

- **380%** no qualification (men)
- **250%** no qualification (women)
- **220%** upper secondary education diploma (men)
- **60%** upper secondary education diploma (women)

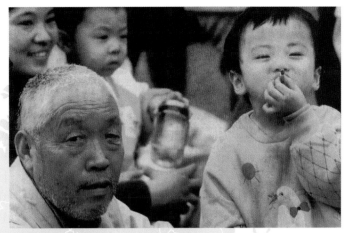

In China, years of education are more important than occupation, income or marital status in relation to cardiovascular risk factors, especially cigarette smoking.

Income and obesity in Saudi Arabia

Percentage of people aged 20 years and above with Body Mass Index of more than 30 kg/m²
1990–1993

income less than US$533	US$ 533–1066	US$ 1067–2133	more than US$2134
22%	19%	24%	28%

Smoking and occupation in Uganda

Percentage of women aged 15 to 54 years and men aged 15 to 59 years who currently smoke daily by category of work
2000–2001

💗 men
💗 women

	agriculture, self-employed	unskilled manual	skilled manual	sales	professional, technical, managerial, clerical	unemployed (previous 12 months)
men	34%	33%	29%	21%	14%	3%
women	4%	3%	2%	1%	0%	2%

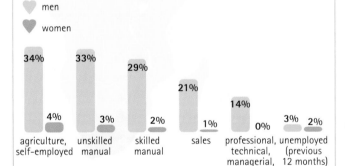
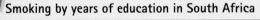

Prevalence of diabetes by income in India

Percentage of people aged 20 years and above with diabetes, by income level
2000

less than US$111	US$ 112–223	more than US$223
13%	19%	22%

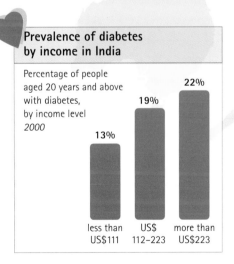

Smoking by years of education in South Africa

Percentage of people aged 15 years and above who currently smoke daily
1998

💗 men
💗 women

	no education	up to 5 years	6–7 years	8–11 years	12 years	more than 12 years
men	45%	45%	39%	35%	33%	25%
women	10%	12%	11%	8%	9%	8%

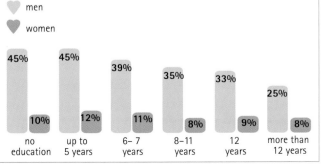

41

Women: a special case?

Widespread misconceptions persist about heart disease, often thought to be primarily a disease of middle-aged men. In reality, cardiovascular disease affects as many women as men, albeit at an older age. Many women still believe that they are more at risk from cancer than from heart disease.

Risk factors for CVD are similar for men and women, but tobacco use is more dangerous in women. In addition, high blood triglycerides are an important cause of atherosclerosis in young women, but not in young men. The menopause has no direct effect, but hormone replacement therapy increases the risk of CVD.

Heart disease is under-detected in women, particularly younger women. In developed countries, women are less likely to be referred to a heart specialist, to be hospitalized, to be prescribed medicine or invasive treatment, or to be referred for exercise testing or echocardiography. Women are more likely to enter the medical system with the diagnosis of a second heart attack.

After a first stroke, women are kept in hospital longer, and remain more disabled than men receiving similar care. More research is needed to improve our understanding of the differences in responses to treatment in men and women.

In the interim, however, adherence to the published guidelines for the prevention and control of heart disease and stroke seems prudent.

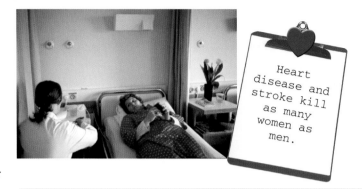

Heart disease and stroke kill as many women as men.

Risk factors

Modifiable risks – risk or prevalence is higher in women than men

- **Tobacco use** (higher risk)
- **High triglyceride levels** (higher risk)
- **Diabetes** (more prevalent)
- **Obesity** (more prevalent)
- **Depression** (more prevalent)

Modifiable risks – risk is similar in men and women

- **High blood pressure**
- **High total cholesterol**
- **Low HDL-cholesterol**
- **Combined hyperlipidaemia**
- **Unhealthy diet**
- **Physical inactivity**
- **Stress**

Risks for women only

- **Oral contraceptive use**
- **Hormone replacement therapy**
- **Polycystic ovary syndrome**
- **Risk of heart attack highest early in each menstrual cycle**

Non-modifiable risks for men and women

- **Advancing age**
- **Gender**
- **Heredity**
- **Ethnicity/race**

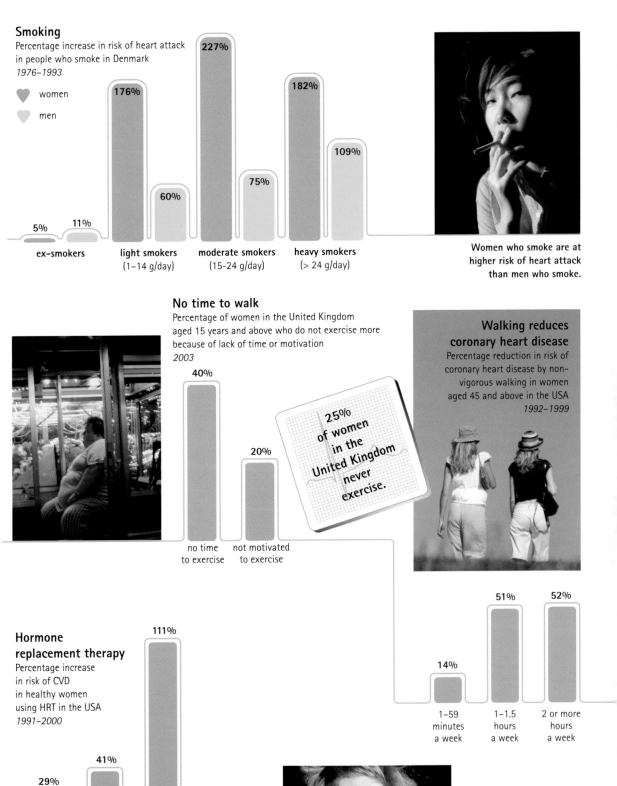

Smoking

Percentage increase in risk of heart attack in people who smoke in Denmark
1976–1993

♥ women

♥ men

5%	11%	227%	182%
		176%	109%
		60%	75%

ex-smokers

light smokers
(1–14 g/day)

moderate smokers
(15–24 g/day)

heavy smokers
(> 24 g/day)

Women who smoke are at higher risk of heart attack than men who smoke.

No time to walk

Percentage of women in the United Kingdom aged 15 years and above who do not exercise more because of lack of time or motivation
2003

40%

20%

no time
to exercise

not motivated
to exercise

25% of women in the United Kingdom never exercise.

Walking reduces coronary heart disease

Percentage reduction in risk of coronary heart disease by non-vigorous walking in women aged 45 and above in the USA
1992–1999

14%

51%

52%

1–59
minutes
a week

1–1.5
hours
a week

2 or more
hours
a week

Hormone replacement therapy

Percentage increase in risk of CVD in healthy women using HRT in the USA
1991–2000

29%

41%

111%

22%

coronary
heart
disease

stroke

deep
venous
thrombosis

all CVD

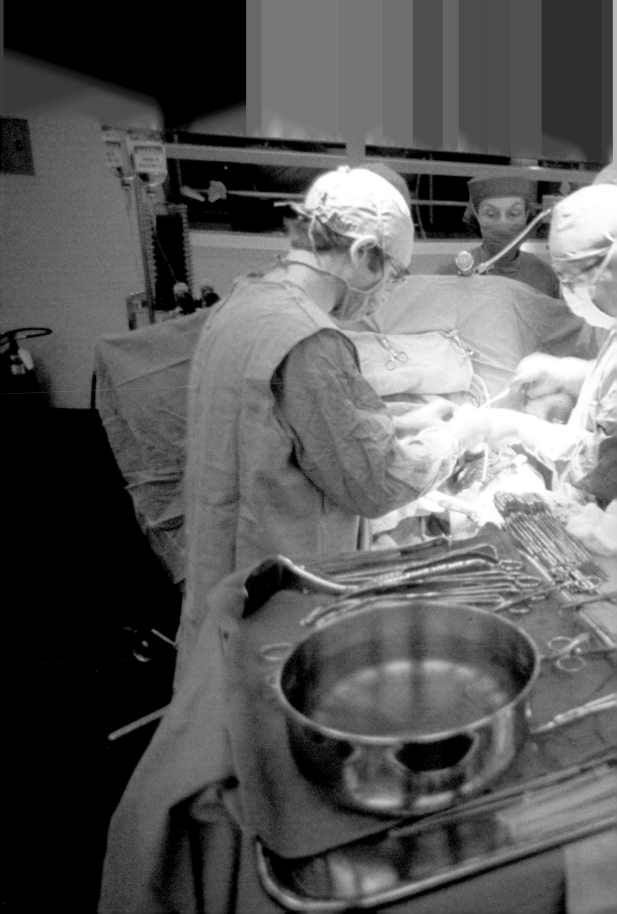

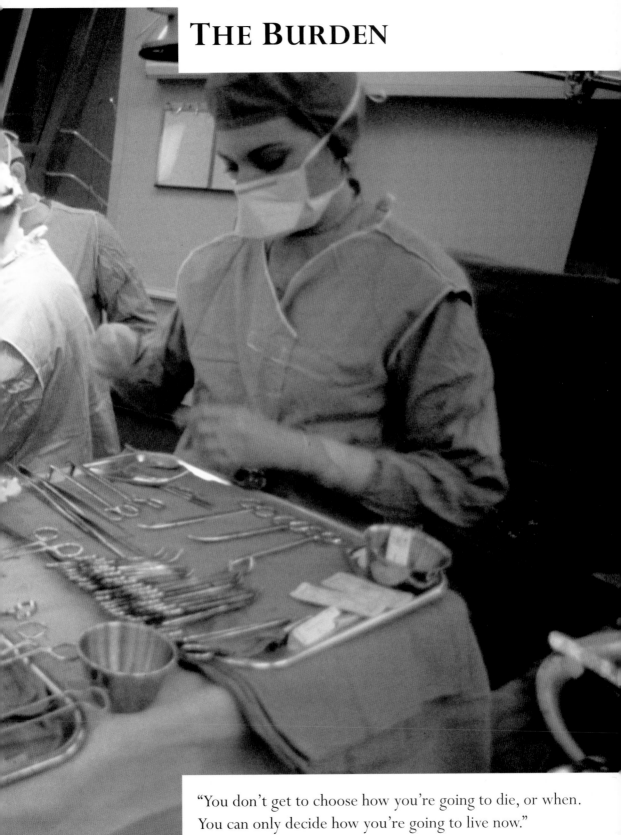

PART 3

THE BURDEN

"You don't get to choose how you're going to die, or when.
You can only decide how you're going to live now."

Joan Baez, folk singer and activist, USA (1941–)

Global burden of coronary heart disease

Disability-adjusted life years (DALYs) lost can be thought of as "healthy years of life lost". They indicate the total burden of a disease, as opposed to simply the resulting deaths.

Cardiovascular disease is responsible for 10% of DALYs lost in low- and middle-income countries, and 18% in high-income countries.

A heart attack occurs when the blood vessels supplying the heart muscle become blocked, starving it of oxygen, leading to the heart muscle's failure or death. Heart attack has the same risk factors as CVD in general. Cold weather, exercise, or strong emotion can precipitate a heart attack.

Coronary heart disease is decreasing in many developed countries, but is increasing in developing and transitional countries, partly as a result of increasing longevity, urbanization, and lifestyle changes.

Risk of heart attack can change when people migrate. Japan has a low rate of coronary heart disease, but after moving to the USA, Japanese people have been found to have a gradually increasing risk. This eventually approaches that of people born in the USA.

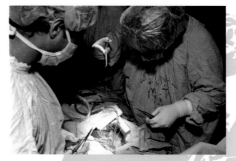

Coronary heart disease burden is projected to rise from around 47 million DALYs globally in 1990 to 82 million DALYs in 2020.

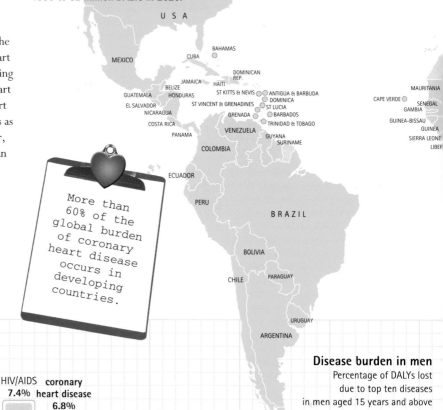

More than 60% of the global burden of coronary heart disease occurs in developing countries.

Disease burden in men
Percentage of DALYs lost due to top ten diseases in men aged 15 years and above
2002

- HIV/AIDS 7.4%
- coronary heart disease 6.8%
- stroke 5.0%
- unipolar depressive disorders 4.8%
- road traffic injuries 4.3%
- tuberculosis 4.2%
- alcohol use disorders 3.4%
- violence 3.3%
- chronic obstructive pulmonary disease 3.1%
- hearing loss, adult 2.7%

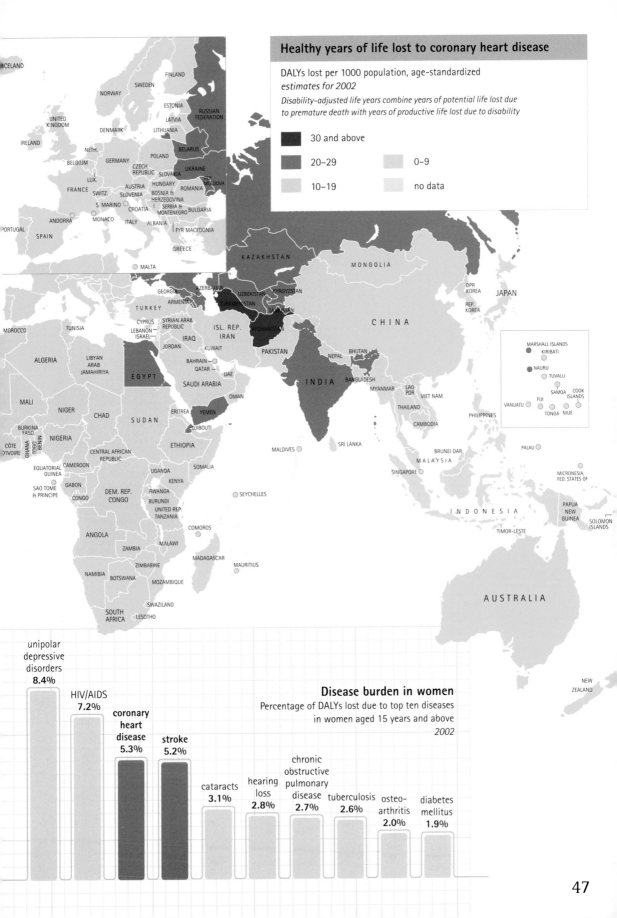

Healthy years of life lost to coronary heart disease

DALYs lost per 1000 population, age-standardized *estimates for 2002*

Disability-adjusted life years combine years of potential life lost due to premature death with years of productive life lost due to disability

- 30 and above
- 20–29
- 10–19
- 0–9
- no data

Disease burden in women

Percentage of DALYs lost due to top ten diseases in women aged 15 years and above
2002

- unipolar depressive disorders **8.4%**
- HIV/AIDS **7.2%**
- coronary heart disease **5.3%**
- stroke **5.2%**
- cataracts **3.1%**
- hearing loss **2.8%**
- chronic obstructive pulmonary disease **2.7%**
- tuberculosis **2.6%**
- osteo-arthritis **2.0%**
- diabetes mellitus **1.9%**

Deaths from coronary heart disease

> "People live with their own idiosyncrasies and die of their own illnesses."
> Vietnamese proverb

Civilization kills. Since 1990, more people have died from coronary heart disease than from any other cause. Unlike stroke, coronary heart disease is a comparative newcomer on the world stage. Variations in death rates are marked: they are lower in populations with short life expectancy.

Heart disease mortality rates are also affected by differences between countries in the major risk factors, especially blood pressure, blood cholesterol, smoking, physical activity and diet. While genetic factors play a part, 80% to 90% of people dying from coronary heart disease have one or more major risk factors that are influenced by lifestyle.

Death rates from coronary heart disease have decreased in North America and many western European countries. This decline has been due to improved prevention, diagnosis, and treatment, in particular reduced cigarette smoking among adults, and lower average levels of blood pressure and blood cholesterol. It is expected that 82% of the future increase in coronary heart disease mortality will occur in developing countries.

Of all coronary heart disease patients who die within 28 days after the onset of symptoms, about two-thirds die before reaching hospital. This highlights not only the need for early recognition of the warning signs of a heart attack, but also the need for prevention.

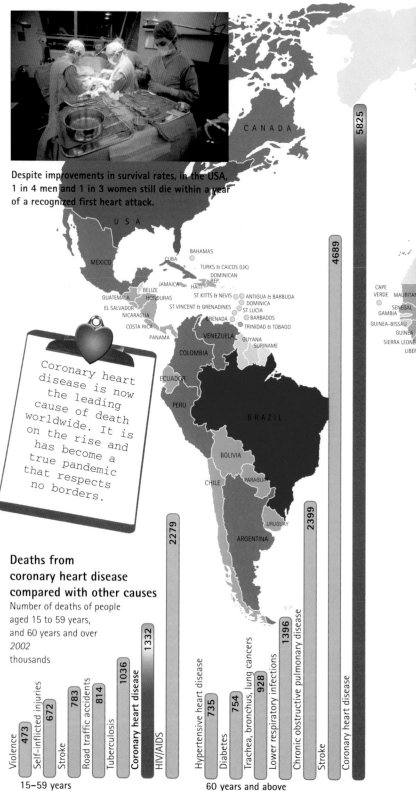

Despite improvements in survival rates, in the USA, 1 in 4 men and 1 in 3 women still die within a year of a recognized first heart attack.

Coronary heart disease is now the leading cause of death worldwide. It is on the rise and has become a true pandemic that respects no borders.

Deaths from coronary heart disease compared with other causes
Number of deaths of people aged 15 to 59 years, and 60 years and over
2002
thousands

15–59 years:
- Violence 473
- Self-inflicted injuries 672
- Stroke 783
- Road traffic accidents 814
- Tuberculosis 1036
- **Coronary heart disease 1332**
- HIV/AIDS 2279

60 years and above:
- Hypertensive heart disease 735
- Diabetes 754
- Trachea, bronchus, lung cancers 928
- Lower respiratory infections 1396
- Chronic obstructive pulmonary disease 2399
- Stroke 4689
- Coronary heart disease 5825

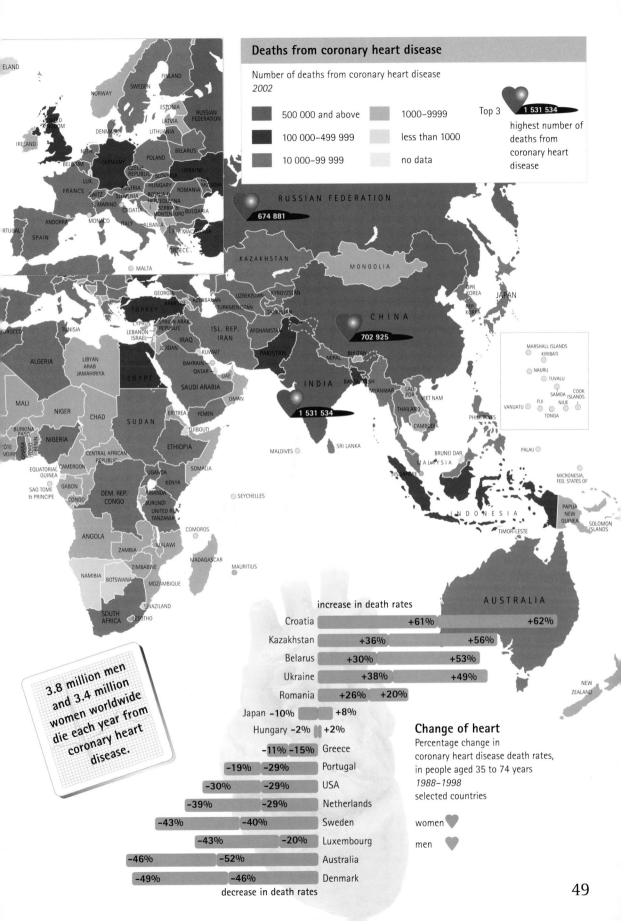

Deaths from coronary heart disease

Number of deaths from coronary heart disease
2002

500 000 and above	1000–9999
100 000–499 999	less than 1000
10 000–99 999	no data

Top 3 **1 531 534**
highest number of deaths from coronary heart disease

RUSSIAN FEDERATION **674 881**

CHINA **702 925**

1 531 534

3.8 million men and 3.4 million women worldwide die each year from coronary heart disease.

increase in death rates

Croatia	+61%	+62%
Kazakhstan	+36%	+56%
Belarus	+30%	+53%
Ukraine	+38%	+49%
Romania	+26%	+20%
Japan	–10%	+8%
Hungary	–2%	+2%
–11%	–15%	Greece
–19%	–29%	Portugal
–30%	–29%	USA
–39%	–29%	Netherlands
–43%	–40%	Sweden
–43%	–20%	Luxembourg
–46%	–52%	Australia
–49%	–46%	Denmark

decrease in death rates

Change of heart
Percentage change in coronary heart disease death rates, in people aged 35 to 74 years
1988–1998
selected countries

women

men

15

"I waked and sat up...when I felt a confusion and indistinctness in my head which lasted, I suppose about half a minute. Soon after I perceived that I had suffered a paralytick stroke, and that my Speech was taken from me."
Samuel Johnson, England, 1783

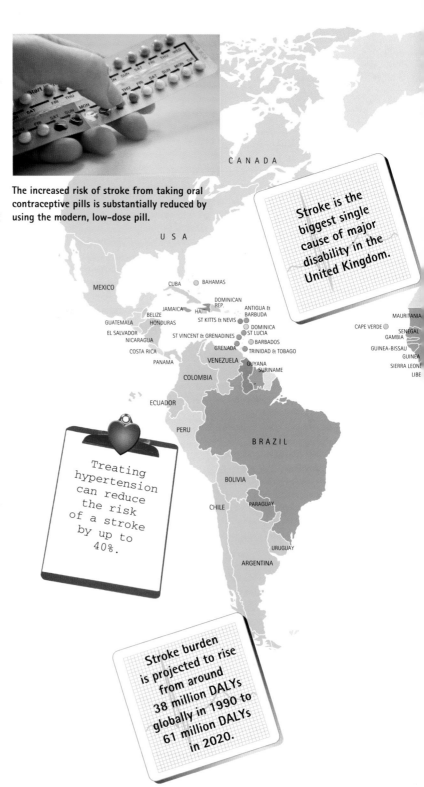

The increased risk of stroke from taking oral contraceptive pills is substantially reduced by using the modern, low-dose pill.

Stroke is the brain equivalent of a heart attack. Blood must flow to and through the brain for it to function. If its flow is obstructed, by a blood clot moving to the brain, or by narrowing or bursting of blood vessels, the brain loses its energy supply, causing damage to tissues leading to stroke.

Annually, 15 million people worldwide suffer a stroke. Of these, 5 million die and another 5 million are left permanently disabled, placing a burden on family and community. Stroke is uncommon in people under 40 years; when it does occur, the main cause is high blood pressure. Stroke also occurs in about 8% of children with sickle cell disease.

The major risk factors for stroke are similar to those for coronary heart disease, with high blood pressure and tobacco use the most significant modifiable risks. Atrial fibrillation, heart failure and heart attack are other important risk factors.

The incidence of stroke is declining in many developed countries, largely as a result of better control of high blood pressure, and reduced levels of smoking. However, the absolute number of strokes continues to increase because of the ageing population.

Stroke is the biggest single cause of major disability in the United Kingdom.

Treating hypertension can reduce the risk of a stroke by up to 40%.

Stroke burden is projected to rise from around 38 million DALYs globally in 1990 to 61 million DALYs in 2020.

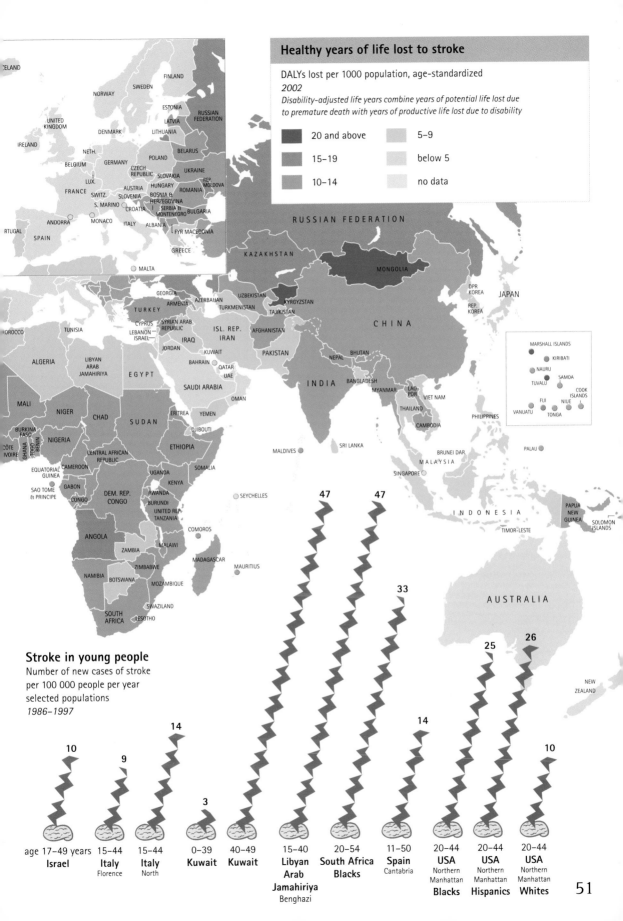

Healthy years of life lost to stroke

DALYs lost per 1000 population, age-standardized
2002
Disability-adjusted life years combine years of potential life lost due to premature death with years of productive life lost due to disability

- 20 and above
- 15–19
- 10–14
- 5–9
- below 5
- no data

Stroke in young people

Number of new cases of stroke per 100 000 people per year selected populations
1986–1997

Value	age	Location
10	age 17–49 years	Israel
9	15–44	Italy Florence
14	15–44	Italy North
3	0–39	Kuwait
47	40–49	Kuwait
47	15–40	Libyan Arab Jamahiriya Benghazi
33	20–54	South Africa Blacks
14	11–50	Spain Cantabria
25	20–44	USA Northern Manhattan Blacks
26	20–44	USA Northern Manhattan Hispanics
10	20–44	USA Northern Manhattan Whites

Stroke carries a high risk of death. Survivors can experience loss of vision and/or speech, paralysis, and confusion. Historically called "apoplexy", "stroke" is so called because of the way it strikes people down.

Previous stroke significantly increases risk of further episodes. Certain racial, ethnic and socioeconomic groups are also at greater risk of stroke. The most important modifiable cause of stroke is high blood pressure; for every ten people who die of stroke, four could have been saved if their blood pressure had been regulated. Among those aged under 65, two-fifths of deaths from stroke are linked to smoking. Other modifiable risk factors include unhealthy diet, high salt intake, underlying heart disease, diabetes and high blood lipids.

The risk of death depends on the type of stroke. Transient ischaemic attack or TIA – where symptoms resolve in less than 24 hours – has the best outcome, followed by stroke caused by carotid stenosis (narrowing of the artery in the neck that supplies blood to the brain). Blockage of an artery is more dangerous, with rupture of a cerebral blood vessel the most dangerous of all.

Even where advanced technology and facilities are available, 60% of those who suffer a stroke die or become dependent. Given these dismal statistics and the high cost of treatment of stroke, high priority should be accorded to preventive strategies.

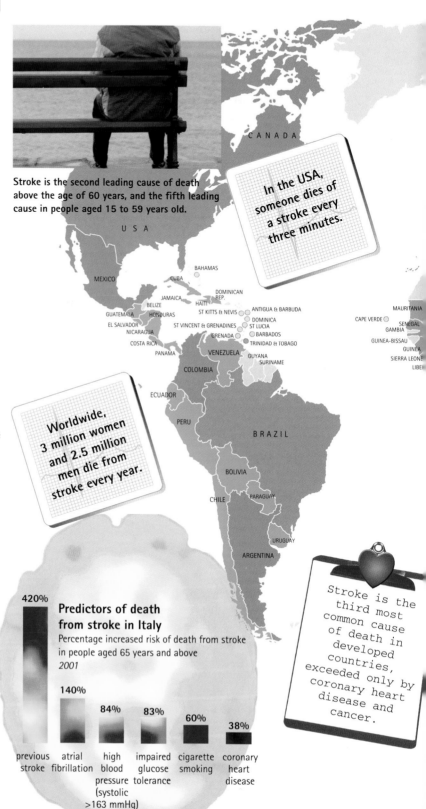

Stroke is the second leading cause of death above the age of 60 years, and the fifth leading cause in people aged 15 to 59 years old.

In the USA, someone dies of a stroke every three minutes.

Worldwide, 3 million women and 2.5 million men die from stroke every year.

Stroke is the third most common cause of death in developed countries, exceeded only by coronary heart disease and cancer.

Predictors of death from stroke in Italy
Percentage increased risk of death from stroke in people aged 65 years and above
2001

previous stroke	atrial fibrillation	high blood pressure (systolic >163 mmHg)	impaired glucose tolerance	cigarette smoking	coronary heart disease
420%	140%	84%	83%	60%	38%

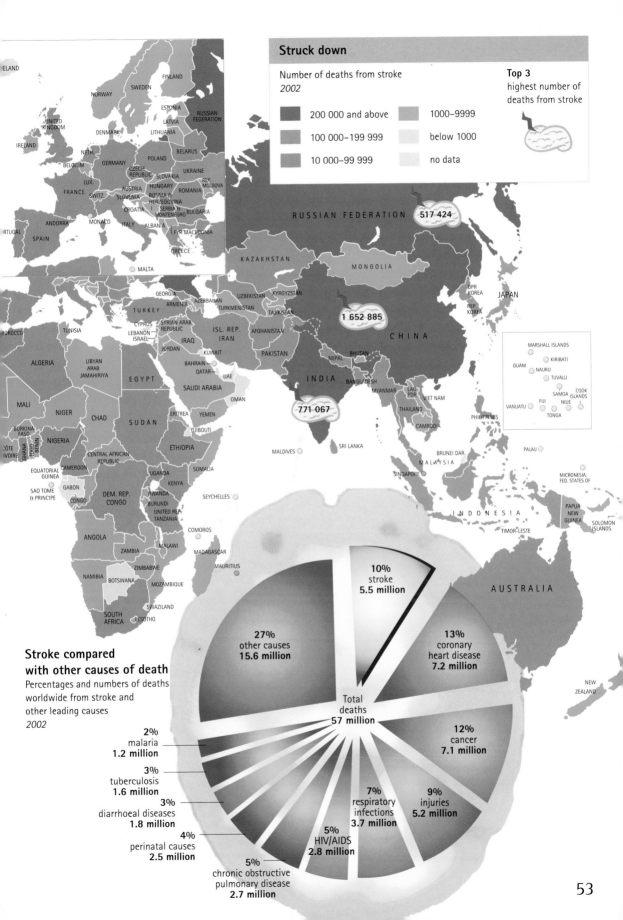

Number of deaths from stroke
2002

200 000 and above	1000–9999
100 000–199 999	below 1000
10 000–99 999	no data

Top 3
highest number of deaths from stroke

RUSSIAN FEDERATION 517 424

1 652 885

771 067

Stroke compared with other causes of death

Percentages and numbers of deaths worldwide from stroke and other leading causes
2002

Total deaths 57 million

10% stroke 5.5 million

13% coronary heart disease 7.2 million

27% other causes 15.6 million

12% cancer 7.1 million

9% injuries 5.2 million

7% respiratory infections 3.7 million

5% HIV/AIDS 2.8 million

5% chronic obstructive pulmonary disease 2.7 million

4% perinatal causes 2.5 million

3% diarrhoeal diseases 1.8 million

3% tuberculosis 1.6 million

2% malaria 1.2 million

53

"The art of economics consists in looking not merely at the immediate but at the longer effects of any act or policy; it consists in tracing the consequences of that policy not merely for one group but for all groups."
Henry Hazlitt, USA (1894–1993)

The costs of cardiovascular disease are diverse: the cost to the individual and to the family of heath care and time off work; the cost to government of health care; and the cost to the country of lost productivity.

We attempt here to quantify some of these costs. However, the value of a human life is beyond our analysis.

Global costs of smoking

Health care costs associated with smoking-related illnesses result in a global net loss of US$200 billion per year, with one third of those losses occurring in developing countries. Estimated 1994.

USA, Australia and Europe

2002 reports indicate that up to 10% of health budgets are spent on diabetes-related illnesses.

USA

"If just 10% of adults began walking regularly, Americans could save US$5.6 billion in costs related to heart disease." – President George W. Bush, 2002.

The direct costs of physical inactivity accounted for an estimated US$24 billion in health care costs in 1995.

Health problems related to obesity, such as heart disease and type 2 diabetes, cost the USA an estimated US$177 billion a year.

Cholesterol reducers were the top-selling medications in 2003, generating US$13.9 billion in sales.

The American Heart Association estimates that stroke will cost a total of US$53.6 billion in 2004. Direct costs for medical care and therapy will average US$33 billion and indirect costs from lost productivity will be US$20.6 billion.

In 2001, the National Stroke Association estimated that the average cost per patient for the first 90 days after a stroke was US$15 000, although 10% of cases cost more than US$35 000.

Latin America and the Caribbean

Permanent disabilities resulting from diabetes cost US$50 billion in 2000, while costs associated with insulin, hospitalization, consultations and care totalled US$10.6 billion.

Global costs of diabetes

Between 4% and 5% of health budgets are spent on diabetes-related illnesses.
WHO, 2003

Price of weekly dose of medication

Expressed in kg of cheapest crop available (yam, rice or potato)
2003
selected countries

Simvastatin
Aspirin

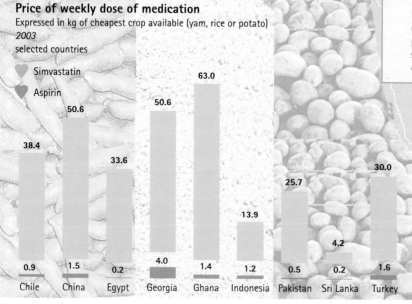

	Chile	China	Egypt	Georgia	Ghana	Indonesia	Pakistan	Sri Lanka	Turkey
Simvastatin	38.4	50.6	33.6	50.6	63.0	13.9	25.7	30.0	
Aspirin	0.9	1.5	0.2	4.0	1.4	1.2	0.5	4.2 / 0.2	1.6

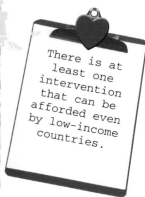

There is at least one intervention that can be afforded even by low-income countries.

United Kingdom

"The direct cost of obesity to the National Health Service is £0.5 billion [about US$0.9 billion] per year, while the indirect cost to the UK economy is at least £2 billion [about US$3.5 billion]."
– Liam Donaldson, Chief Medical Officer, 2003

More than 4% of National Health Service spending was on stroke services in 2000.

The economics of CVD

 physical exercise   stroke   diabetes

obesity   CVD

cholesterol   tobacco

Netherlands

The average total costs of care per patient for six months following a stroke were estimated at €16 000 in 2003.

Stroke was estimated to be responsible for 3% of total health care costs in the Netherlands in 1994, and 7% of costs for the population aged 75 and over. Stroke ranked second on the list of most costly diseases for the elderly, after dementia, and these costs are expected to increase by 40% by 2015.

Global costs of heart disease medication

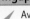
The number of people who die or are disabled by coronary heart disease and stroke could be halved with wider use of a combination of drugs that costs just US$14 a year.
WHO, 2002

Singapore

Average hospital costs for stroke were reported in 2000 as US$5000 per patient. Ward charges accounted for 38%, radiology 15%, doctors' fees 10%, medications 8%, therapy 7%.

The cost of risk factors

Cumulative Medicare costs of treatment of cardiovascular disease in people aged 65 years to death, in the USA
2000
US$

Risk factors:
high blood pressure, high cholesterol, cigarette smoking, abnormal electrocardiograms, a history of diabetes or previous heart attacks

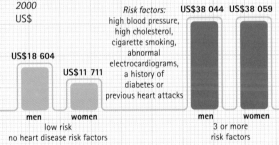

US$18 604 — men — low risk no heart disease risk factors
US$11 711 — women — low risk no heart disease risk factors
US$38 044 — men — 3 or more risk factors
US$38 059 — women — 3 or more risk factors

Lifetime costs of coronary heart disease

Germany
1996
US$

US$26 billion — Total direct costs
Including: primary care, clinical care, rehabilitation

US$48 billion — Total indirect costs
Lost productivity caused by: short-term and long-term disability, death

Average cost per case: US$82 000

Expenditure on cardiovascular medications

Percentage of total annual drug expenditure
1989–1997
OECD countries

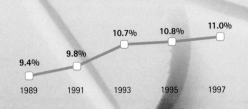

9.4% (1989)   9.8% (1991)   10.7% (1993)   10.8% (1995)   11.0% (1997)

Aspirin remains the least expensive drug for secondary prevention.

55

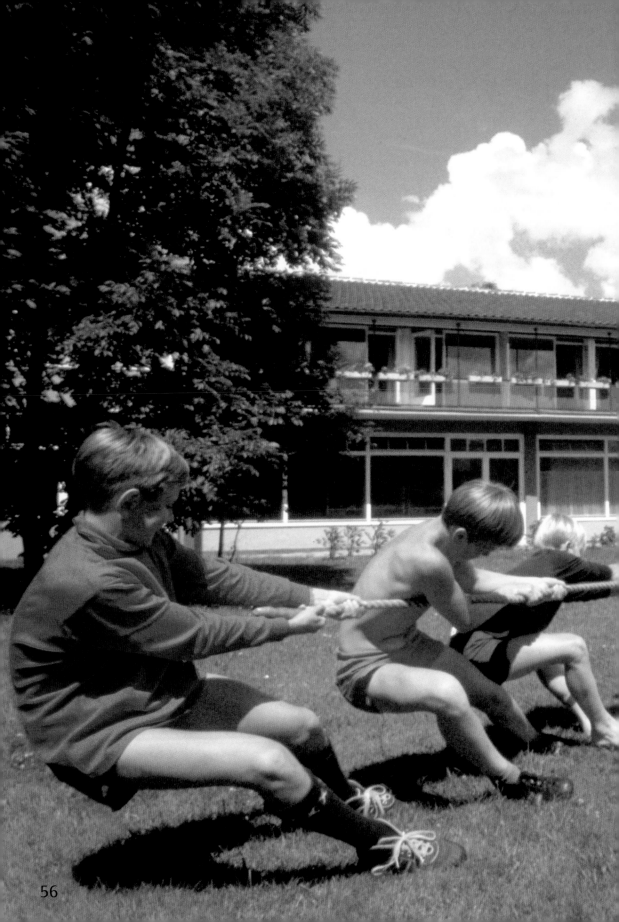

PART 4

ACTION

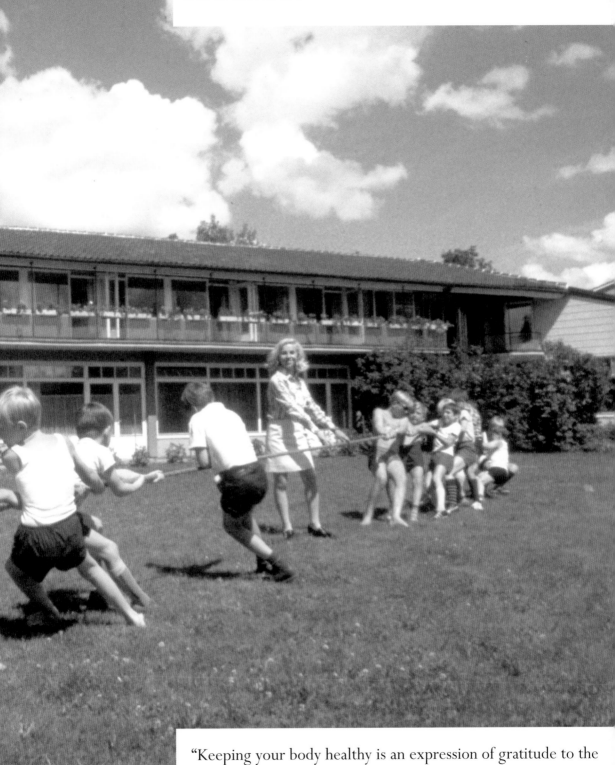

"Keeping your body healthy is an expression of gratitude to the whole cosmos, the trees, the clouds, everything."

Most Venerable Thich Nhat Hanh, Vietnamese Buddhist monk (1926–)

Research

> "Science knows no country, because knowledge belongs to humanity, and is the torch that illuminates the world."
> Louis Pasteur, France (1822–1892)

From the description of how a heart muscle cell contracts to the elucidation of the human genome, scientific advances in basic, clinical, and population research in cardiovascular disease, and their global impact, have been phenomenal. New and improved treatments have become possible, and novel markers of future risk have been identified.

Yet several key challenges remain. There is a widespread lack of research capacity, standardized data, communication networks, and human and financial resources, especially in developing countries.

The MONICA (Multinational MONItoring of trends and determinants in CArdiovascular disease) Project involved teams from 38 populations in 21 countries from the mid-1980s to the mid-1990s, the largest such collaboration ever undertaken. It was set up to explain the diverse trends in cardiovascular disease mortality observed from the 1970s onwards. The project monitored a study population of 10 million men and women, aged 25 to 64 years.

MONICA was important in measuring levels and trends in cardiovascular diseases and their risk factors in different populations, in monitoring prevention policies in different countries, and in demonstrating the importance of the new acute and long-term treatments that were being introduced.

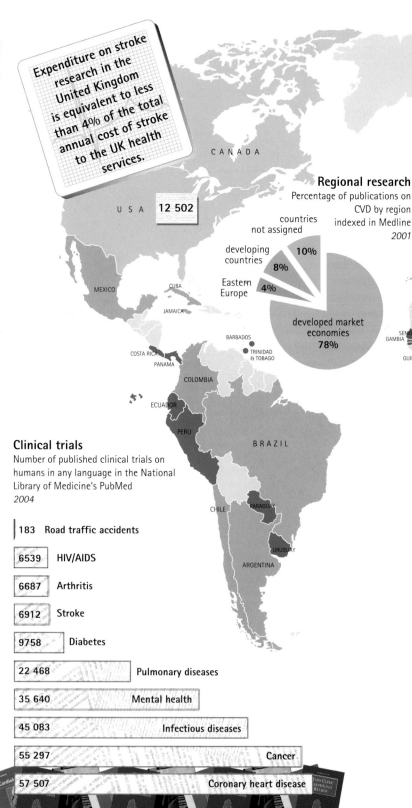

Expenditure on stroke research in the United Kingdom is equivalent to less than 4% of the total annual cost of stroke to the UK health services.

Regional research
Percentage of publications on CVD by region indexed in Medline
2001

- countries not assigned **10%**
- developing countries **8%**
- Eastern Europe **4%**
- developed market economies **78%**

Clinical trials
Number of published clinical trials on humans in any language in the National Library of Medicine's PubMed
2004

183	Road traffic accidents
6539	HIV/AIDS
6687	Arthritis
6912	Stroke
9758	Diabetes
22 468	Pulmonary diseases
35 640	Mental health
45 083	Infectious diseases
55 297	Cancer
57 507	Coronary heart disease

USA **12 502**

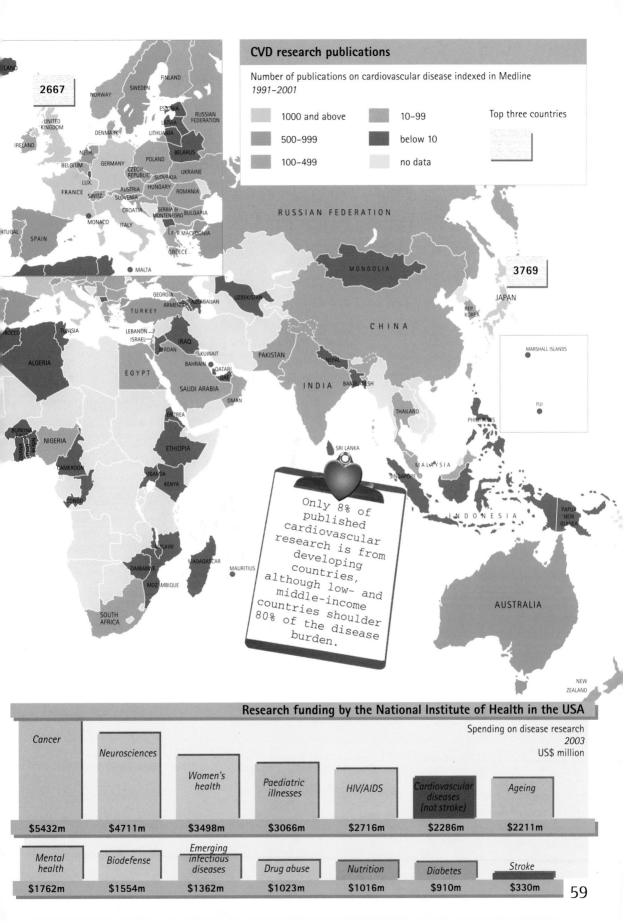

CVD research publications

Number of publications on cardiovascular disease indexed in Medline
1991–2001

- 1000 and above
- 500–999
- 100–499
- 10–99
- below 10
- no data

Top three countries

2667

3769

> Only 8% of published cardiovascular research is from developing countries, although low- and middle-income countries shoulder 80% of the disease burden.

Research funding by the National Institute of Health in the USA

Spending on disease research
2003
US$ million

Cancer	Neurosciences	Women's health	Paediatric illnesses	HIV/AIDS	Cardiovascular diseases (not stroke)	Ageing
$5432m	$4711m	$3498m	$3066m	$2716m	$2286m	$2211m

Mental health	Biodefense	Emerging infectious diseases	Drug abuse	Nutrition	Diabetes	Stroke
$1762m	$1554m	$1362m	$1023m	$1016m	$910m	$330m

59

> "Don't agonize. Organize."
> Florynce Kennedy, Lawyer, and Civil and
> Womens' Rights Activist (1916–2000)

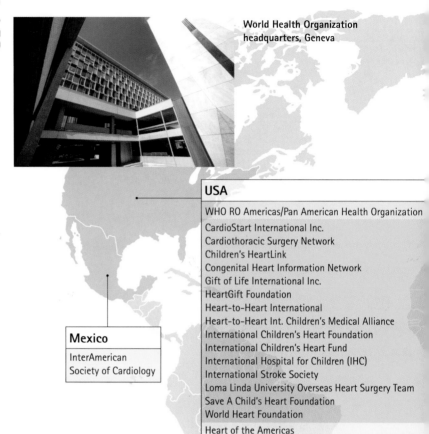

World Health Organization
headquarters, Geneva

The World Health Organization's Cardiovascular Disease Programme is conducted through its Geneva headquarters, and regional and national offices worldwide. The World Heart Federation helps people achieve a longer, better life through prevention and control of heart disease and stroke, focusing on low- and middle-income countries.

In addition to the nongovernmental organizations (NGOs) highlighted here, there are many international NGOs – from the World Medical Association to Consumers International – that include cardiovascular disease control as part of their activities.

Only international and regional organizations are shown here. Not mentioned are the many national organizations, whose impact may extend outside their own country, such as the Centers for Disease Control and Prevention in the USA, the British Heart Foundation, and ThaiHealth in Thailand. Other national NGOs also work part time on CVD issues.

There are numerous other partners in a vast arena of varied but related interests, including organizations involved with women, youth, law, economics, human rights, religion and development.

The capacity of virtually all cardiovascular disease control organizations is inadequate to meet the challenge of the CVD epidemic.

Mexico

InterAmerican
Society of Cardiology

USA

WHO RO Americas/Pan American Health Organization
CardioStart International Inc.
Cardiothoracic Surgery Network
Children's HeartLink
Congenital Heart Information Network
Gift of Life International Inc.
HeartGift Foundation
Heart-to-Heart International
Heart-to-Heart Int. Children's Medical Alliance
International Children's Heart Foundation
International Children's Heart Fund
International Hospital for Children (IHC)
International Stroke Society
Loma Linda University Overseas Heart Surgery Team
Save A Child's Heart Foundation
World Heart Foundation

Heart of the Americas
InterAmerican Heart Foundation

World Conferences on Cardiovascular Diseases

World Congresses of Cardiology		
1st	1974	Buenos Aires, Argentina
2nd	1978	Tokyo, Japan
3rd	1982	Moscow, Russian Federation
4th	1986	Washington, DC, USA
5th	1990	Manila, Philippines
6th	1994	Berlin, Germany
7th	1998	Rio de Janeiro, Brazil
8th	2002	Sydney, Australia
9th	2006	Barcelona, Spain

International Conferences on Preventive Cardiology		
1st	1985	Moscow, USSR
2nd	1989	Washington, DC, USA
3rd	1993	Oslo, Norway
4th	1997	Montreal, Canada
5th	2001	Osaka, Japan
6th	2005	Iguassu, Brazil

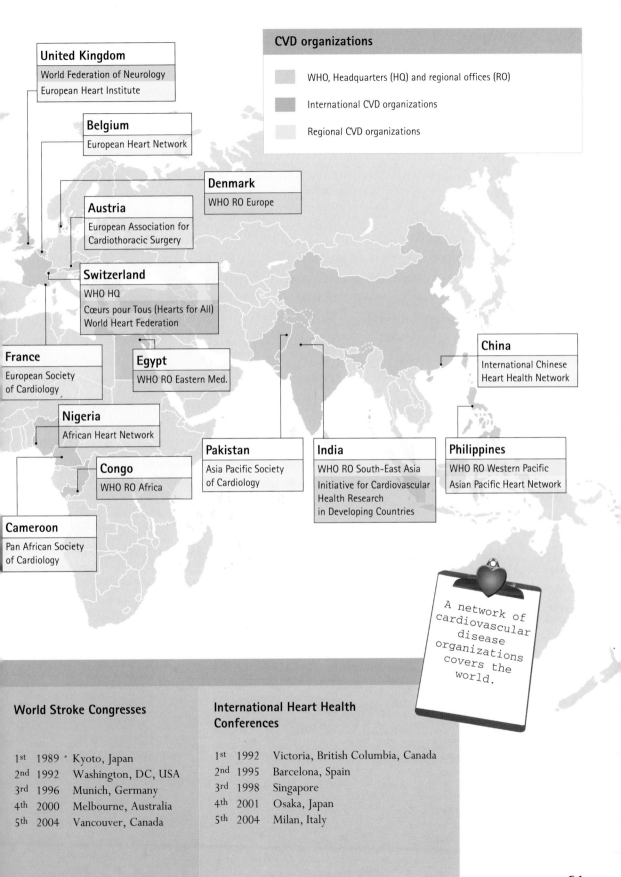

CVD organizations

WHO, Headquarters (HQ) and regional offices (RO)

International CVD organizations

Regional CVD organizations

United Kingdom
World Federation of Neurology
European Heart Institute

Belgium
European Heart Network

Denmark
WHO RO Europe

Austria
European Association for
Cardiothoracic Surgery

Switzerland
WHO HQ
Cœurs pour Tous (Hearts for All)
World Heart Federation

China
International Chinese
Heart Health Network

France
European Society
of Cardiology

Egypt
WHO RO Eastern Med.

Nigeria
African Heart Network

Pakistan
Asia Pacific Society
of Cardiology

Congo
WHO RO Africa

India
WHO RO South-East Asia
Initiative for Cardiovascular
Health Research
in Developing Countries

Philippines
WHO RO Western Pacific
Asian Pacific Heart Network

Cameroon
Pan African Society
of Cardiology

A network of
cardiovascular
disease
organizations
covers the
world.

World Stroke Congresses

1st 1989   Kyoto, Japan
2nd 1992   Washington, DC, USA
3rd 1996   Munich, Germany
4th 2000   Melbourne, Australia
5th 2004   Vancouver, Canada

**International Heart Health
Conferences**

1st 1992   Victoria, British Columbia, Canada
2nd 1995   Barcelona, Spain
3rd 1998   Singapore
4th 2001   Osaka, Japan
5th 2004   Milan, Italy

61

20 | Prevention: personal choices and actions

> "No matter how far you have gone
> on the wrong road, turn back."
> **Turkish proverb**

Good control of blood pressure, blood cholesterol and blood sugar levels, and other cardiovascular risk factors is the key to reducing risks of heart disease and stroke.

Personal behaviour and lifestyle choices can make a big difference to the risk of coronary heart disease and stroke. It is estimated that having a high-risk lifestyle may account for 82% of coronary events in women. Here, we identify personal choices that can lower individual risk for heart disease and stroke. The choices apply to young people and adults alike.

Personal choices in lifestyles and behaviour

1 Take moderate physical activity for a total of 30 minutes on most days of the week.

2 Avoid tobacco use and exposure to environmental smoke; make plans to quit if you already smoke.

3 Choose a diet rich in fruits, vegetables and potassium, and avoid saturated fats and calorie-dense meals.

4 Maintain a normal body weight; if you are overweight, lose weight by increasing physical activity and reducing calorie intake.

5 Reduce stress at home and at work.

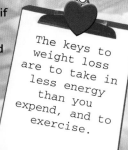

The keys to weight loss are to take in less energy than you expend, and to exercise.

Personal actions for safeguarding cardiovascular health

1 Discuss all questions with your health care provider.

2 Have regular check-ups from your health care provider.

3 Have your blood pressure and levels of blood sugar and cholesterol checked.

4 Follow your health care provider's instructions regarding physical activity, nutrition, weight management, and any medications you have been prescribed.

5 Know the signs and symptoms of heart attack and stroke and remember that both conditions are medical emergencies.

6 Know your blood pressure and cholesterol level, and keep them at the recommended levels through lifestyle changes and by taking any prescribed medication.

7 Lower your total fat and saturated fat intake in accordance with your health care provider's instructions.

For people with diabetes, blood pressure control reduces cardio-vascular disease significantly more than close control of blood sugar

Talk to your health care provider before taking any drugs, including aspirin, to prevent heart disease and stroke.

Young people

1 Actions and choices for children and adolescents with cardiovascular disease, or risk factors, should be discussed with a paediatrician or health care provider.

2 Choose a diet containing a variety of fruits, vegetables, whole grains, dairy products, fish, legumes, poultry, and lean meat.

3 There is no need to restrict fat intake in children under two years of age.

4 For children over two years and adolescents, limit foods high in saturated fats (to less than 10% of daily calorie intake), cholesterol (to less than 300 mg per day), and trans-fatty acids.

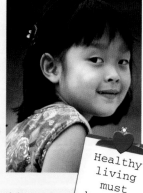

Healthy living must begin in childhood and youth.

5 Increase physical activity, and avoid tobacco use or exposure to environmental tobacco smoke.

Eat fruit and cereals

Percentage reduction in risk
with each daily increment of 10 g of dietary fibre
reported 2004

all coronary events

coronary deaths

Fibre intake

14% 27% 10% 25% 16% 30%

total dietary fibre　　　cereal　　　fruit

In the USA, people eat twice as much sugar and fat as recommended.

Burning calories through physical activity is as important as watching what you eat.

In Japan, since the 1970s, the "10 000 Steps Project" has set a national daily exercise goal. To monitor steps walked, the average Japanese family today owns three pedometers.

Compared with less active people, moderately active and highly active individuals have a 20% and 27% respectively lower risk of stroke or stroke death.

People with low fitness are up to six times more likely to develop diabetes and high blood pressure.

The benefits of stopping smoking

Time since last cigarette	Effect
20 minutes	Blood pressure and pulse rate drop to normal.
1 day	Probability of heart attack begins to decrease.
3 months	Circulation improves.
1 year	Excess risk of coronary heart disease is half that of a continuing smoker.
5 to 15 years later	Risk of stroke is reduced to that of people who have never smoked.
15 years later	Risk of coronary heart disease is similar to that of people who have never smoked, and the overall risk of death almost the same, especially if the smoker quits before illness develops.

Prevention: population and systems approaches

Significant health gains in cardiovascular health can be made within short time spans, through public health and treatment interventions that have an impact on large segments of the population.

As shown here, there is a gap between what is known and what is done in practice, for both prevention and treatment of cardiovascular disease.

Governments are stewards of health resources, and have a fundamental responsibility to protect the health of citizens. Ministries of Health and the health profession can play various roles in reducing CVD, by making data available, educating the public, making treatments affordable and available, advising patients on healthy living practices, and advocating for policy and environmental change. These have been the essential messages of the International Heart Health Conferences and the related declarations on heart health.

Noncommunicable disease (NCD) prevention and control
Percentage of countries with integration of components of NCD prevention and control programmes in primary health care
2001
WHO regions

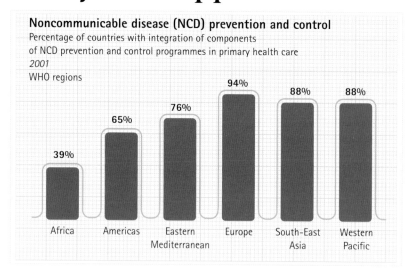

- Africa: 39%
- Americas: 65%
- Eastern Mediterranean: 76%
- Europe: 94%
- South-East Asia: 88%
- Western Pacific: 88%

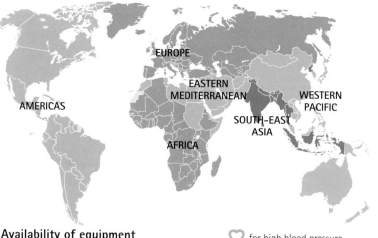

EUROPE
EASTERN MEDITERRANEAN
WESTERN PACIFIC
AMERICAS
SOUTH-EAST ASIA
AFRICA

Availability of equipment
Percentage availability of basic equipment at primary health care level for diagnosis and management of high blood pressure and diabetes
2001
WHO regions

♡ for high blood pressure
♡ for diabetes

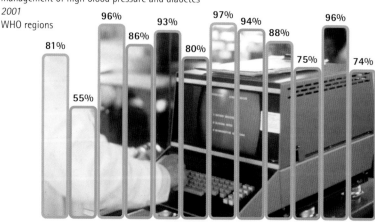

- Africa: 81%, 55%
- Americas: 96%, 86%
- Eastern Mediterranean: 93%, 80%
- Europe: 97%, 94%
- South-East Asia: 88%, 75%
- Western Pacific: 96%, 74%

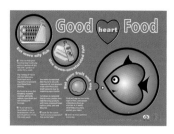

UK dieticians promote the benefits for heart health of eating oily fish, more fruit and vegetables, and less saturated fat.

Medical professionals

Number of medical professionals working in noncommunicable disease control per 100 000 population
2001
WHO regions

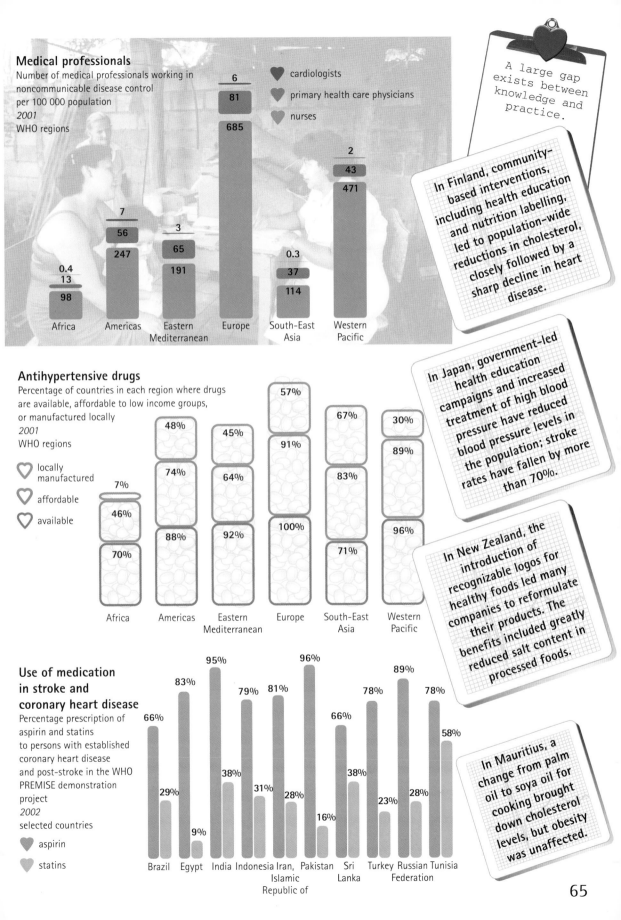

- cardiologists
- primary health care physicians
- nurses

Region	cardiologists	primary health care physicians	nurses
Africa	0.4	13	98
Americas	7	56	247
Eastern Mediterranean	3	65	191
Europe	6	81	685
South-East Asia	0.3	37	114
Western Pacific	2	43	471

Antihypertensive drugs

Percentage of countries in each region where drugs are available, affordable to low income groups, or manufactured locally
2001
WHO regions

- locally manufactured
- affordable
- available

Region	locally manufactured	affordable	available
Africa	7%	46%	70%
Americas	48%	74%	88%
Eastern Mediterranean	45%	64%	92%
Europe	57%	91%	100%
South-East Asia	67%	83%	71%
Western Pacific	30%	89%	96%

Use of medication in stroke and coronary heart disease

Percentage prescription of aspirin and statins to persons with established coronary heart disease and post-stroke in the WHO PREMISE demonstration project
2002
selected countries

- aspirin
- statins

Country	aspirin	statins
Brazil	66%	29%
Egypt	83%	9%
India	95%	38%
Indonesia	79%	31%
Iran, Islamic Republic of	81%	28%
Pakistan	96%	16%
Sri Lanka	66%	38%
Turkey	78%	23%
Russian Federation	89%	28%
Tunisia	78%	58%

A large gap exists between knowledge and practice.

In Finland, community-based interventions, including health education and nutrition labelling, led to population-wide reductions in cholesterol, closely followed by a sharp decline in heart disease.

In Japan, government-led health education campaigns and increased treatment of high blood pressure have reduced blood pressure levels in the population; stroke rates have fallen by more than 70%.

In New Zealand, the introduction of recognizable logos for healthy foods led many companies to reformulate their products. The benefits included greatly reduced salt content in processed foods.

In Mauritius, a change from palm oil to soya oil for cooking brought down cholesterol levels, but obesity was unaffected.

Health education

> "Education is the most powerful weapon which you can use to change the world."
> Nelson Mandela, South Africa (1918-)

For successful prevention and control of the cardiovascular disease epidemic, changes to policy, legislation and taxation are not enough. These interventions will not be effective if there is no public understanding, support and demand for them. Some areas lie beyond legislation – for example, the choice of food for families, the amount of salt added in cooking, whether or not to smoke – and here health education is essential to promote healthy choices.

Schools provide an ideal venue for health education. They can teach about risk factors, refusal skills, and the strategies of the tobacco and food industries. For example, young people can analyse how tobacco industry promotion attempts to manipulate them by equating smoking with growing up, freedom and being cool.

Increasing knowledge, and changing beliefs, attitudes and intentions, on their own are not enough to change behaviour. School programmes must also lead by example, by making healthy food available, providing exercise facilities, prohibiting tobacco use at all school facilities and events, and helping students and staff lose weight and quit smoking. Ideally, these activities should be part of a coordinated school health programme, reinforced by community-wide efforts.

The WHO Global School Health Initiative is designed to strengthen international, national and local support for effective school health programmes or "health-promoting schools". Guidelines have been developed on various factors that affect health, such as tobacco, diet and physical activity.

The WHO Global School-based Student Health Survey is aimed at adolescents aged 13 to 15 years, and covers nine risk or protective factors. Survey results will provide information on trends over time, which is useful for formulation of risk reduction policies.

World Heart Day

World Heart Federation event

▨ participating countries and territories *2003*

Heart Health Declarations

See Milestones pp76-81 for further details

1992 Canada
The Victoria Declaration on Heart Health

2000 Canada
The Victoria Declaration on Women, Heart Disease and Stroke

World Heart Day Themes

- **2000 Physical Activity**
- **2001 A Heart for Life**
- **2002 Nutrition and Physical Activity**

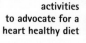

- **2003 Women, Heart Disease and Stroke**
- **2004 Children, Adolescents and Heart Disease**
- **2005 Obesity**

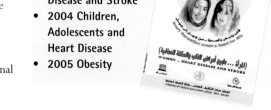

World Heart Day Activities *2001*

medical activities (e.g. blood pressure testing)	**68.5%** of countries
activities to engage the public in physical activity	**65%** of countries
scientific activities (e.g. conferences or workshops)	**61%** of countries
activities to advocate for a heart healthy diet	**35%** of countries
other activities (e.g. charity gala, dance, concert, carnival)	**35%** of countries

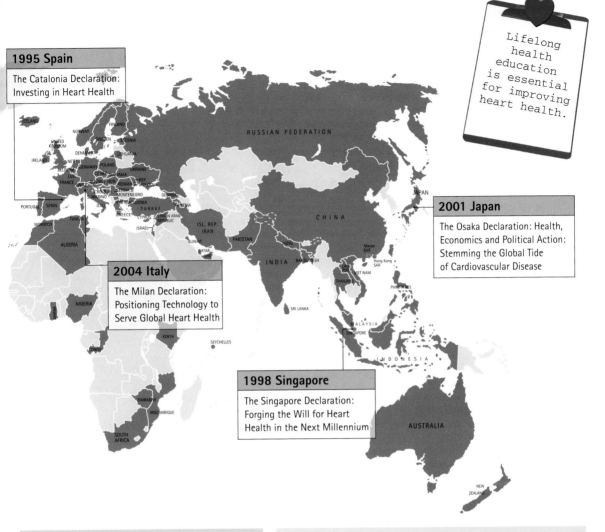

1995 Spain

The Catalonia Declaration:
Investing in Heart Health

Lifelong
health
education
is essential
for improving
heart health.

2001 Japan

The Osaka Declaration: Health,
Economics and Political Action:
Stemming the Global Tide
of Cardiovascular Disease

2004 Italy

The Milan Declaration:
Positioning Technology to
Serve Global Heart Health

1998 Singapore

The Singapore Declaration:
Forging the Will for Heart
Health in the Next Millennium

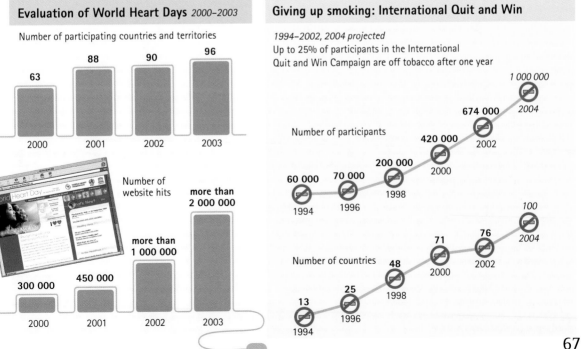

Evaluation of World Heart Days *2000–2003*

Number of participating countries and territories

63	88	90	96
2000	2001	2002	2003

Number of
website hits

300 000	450 000	more than 1 000 000	more than 2 000 000
2000	2001	2002	2003

Giving up smoking: International Quit and Win

1994–2002, 2004 projected
Up to 25% of participants in the International
Quit and Win Campaign are off tobacco after one year

Number of participants

1 000 000 *2004*
674 000 *2004*
420 000 *2002*
200 000 *2000*
60 000 *1994*
70 000 *1996*
1998

Number of countries

100 *2004*
76 *2004*
71 *2002*
48 *2000*
25 *1998*
13 *1994*
1996

67

Laws, treaties, policies and
regulations have played important
roles in the prevention and
control of disease. Only
governments can legislate for
health warnings on cigarettes,
introduce mandatory food
standards and labelling, crack
down on smuggling, set a "pro-
health tax policy", or implement
national transport policy. Often
governments are the main
providers of health care; they
decide how funding is allocated,
from prevention programmes to
treatment, research, and training.

The first international
convention that relates specifically
to cardiovascular disease is the
WHO Framework Convention on
Tobacco Control. It was adopted
without dissent by the World
Health Assembly in Geneva in
May 2003, and is currently in the
process of ratification. Once
40 countries have ratified the
Convention, it will come into
effect as a legally binding treaty
among those countries. The
Convention includes clauses on
advertising bans, smoke-free
areas, health warnings, taxation,
smoking cessation and smuggling.

17th century:
earliest
known bans
on smoking
enacted.

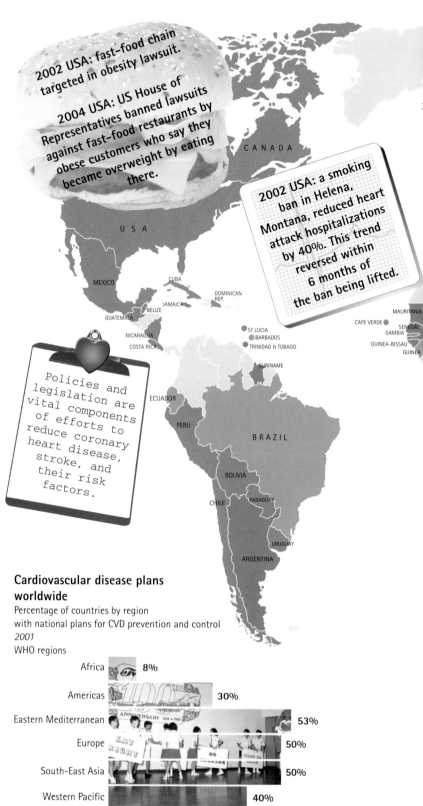

2002 USA: fast-food chain
targeted in obesity lawsuit.

2004 USA: US House of
Representatives banned lawsuits
against fast-food restaurants by
obese customers who say they
became overweight by eating
there.

2002 USA: a smoking
ban in Helena,
Montana, reduced heart
attack hospitalizations
by 40%. This trend
reversed within
6 months of
the ban being lifted.

Policies and
legislation are
vital components
of efforts to
reduce coronary
heart disease,
stroke, and
their risk
factors.

Cardiovascular disease plans worldwide

Percentage of countries by region
with national plans for CVD prevention and control
2001
WHO regions

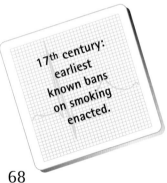

Region	
Africa	8%
Americas	30%
Eastern Mediterranean	53%
Europe	50%
South-East Asia	50%
Western Pacific	40%

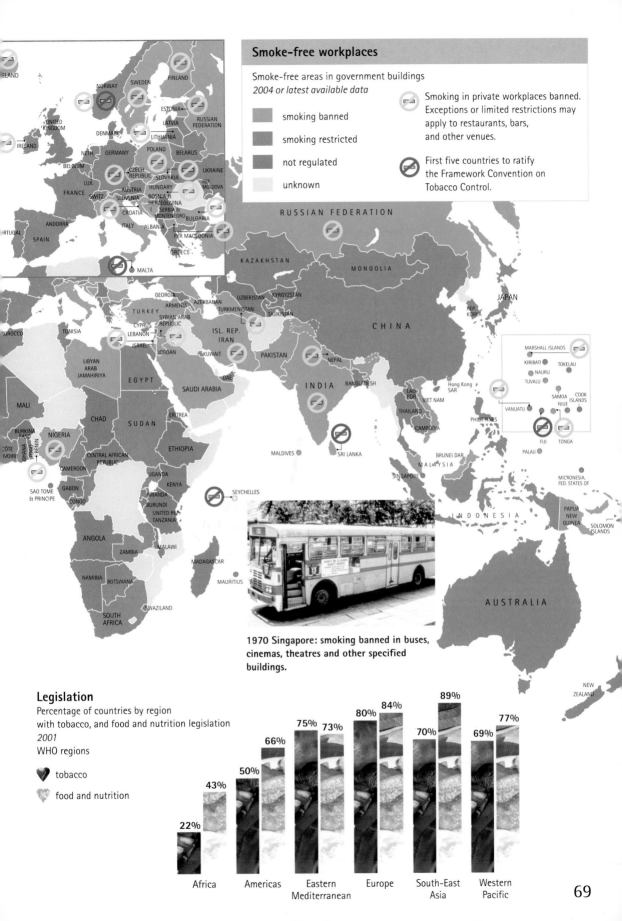

Smoke-free workplaces

Smoke-free areas in government buildings
2004 or latest available data

- smoking banned
- smoking restricted
- not regulated
- unknown

Smoking in private workplaces banned. Exceptions or limited restrictions may apply to restaurants, bars, and other venues.

First five countries to ratify the Framework Convention on Tobacco Control.

1970 Singapore: smoking banned in buses, cinemas, theatres and other specified buildings.

Legislation

Percentage of countries by region with tobacco, and food and nutrition legislation
2001
WHO regions

♥ tobacco
♥ food and nutrition

Region	tobacco	food and nutrition
Africa	22%	43%
Americas	50%	66%
Eastern Mediterranean	75%	73%
Europe	80%	84%
South-East Asia	89%	70%
Western Pacific	69%	77%

"If you do not repair your gutter, you will have your whole house to repair."
Old Spanish proverb

In 1931, Paul Dudley White noted that there was no specific treatment for coronary heart disease. He described the treatment of high blood pressure as "difficult and almost hopeless". Today, effective and relatively inexpensive medication is available to treat nearly all cardiovascular diseases, including high blood pressure.

Improvements in surgical techniques have led to safer operations. Effective devices have been developed, such as pacemakers, prosthetic valves, and patches for closing holes in the heart. Other developments have led to a wide array of interventions that often make surgery unnecessary.

Together, these advances in treatment improve quality of life and reduce premature death and disability. They also add to the rising costs of health care. Increasingly, high-technology procedures are chosen over less expensive, but nevertheless effective, strategies.

In addition, marked disparities in the quality of treatment can be seen in groups of different race, ethnicity, sex, and socioeconomic status. In essence, many patients who could benefit from treatment remain untreated, or inadequately treated. In future, increased emphasis needs to be placed on the appropriate use of proven treatments for everyone with coronary heart disease or stroke.

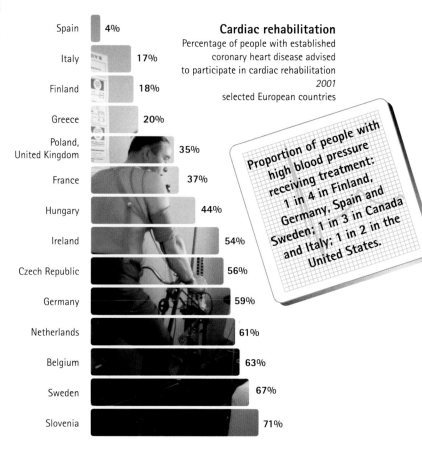

Cardiac rehabilitation
Percentage of people with established coronary heart disease advised to participate in cardiac rehabilitation
2001
selected European countries

Country	Percentage
Spain	4%
Italy	17%
Finland	18%
Greece	20%
Poland, United Kingdom	35%
France	37%
Hungary	44%
Ireland	54%
Czech Republic	56%
Germany	59%
Netherlands	61%
Belgium	63%
Sweden	67%
Slovenia	71%

Proportion of people with high blood pressure receiving treatment: 1 in 4 in Finland, Germany, Spain and Sweden; 1 in 3 in Canada and Italy; 1 in 2 in the United States.

Patients reaching blood pressure and blood cholesterol goals during treatment
Percentage of people aged 70 years or below with established CVD who achieve blood pressure goal of less than 140/90 mmHg, or blood cholesterol goal of less than 5.0 mmol/l
2001
selected European countries

♥ blood cholesterol goal achieved
♥ blood pressure goal achieved

Country	Cholesterol	Blood pressure
Belgium	23%	55%
Czech Republic	28%	57%
Finland	57%	50%
France	40%	44%
Germany	34%	36%
Greece	36%	52%
Hungary	40%	63%
Ireland	46%	50%
Italy	43%	51%
Netherlands	56%	49%
Poland	36%	52%
Slovenia	32%	38%
Spain	60%	36%
Sweden	47%	55%
United Kingdom	47%	49%

Types of treatment

Selected medication, devices and operations

Medication used in treatment of

1 High blood pressure

2 Coronary heart disease

3 Heart failure

4 Arrhythmia (heart rhythm disorders)

5 Blood clotting disorders

Devices

1 Pacemakers

2 Implantable defibrillators

3 Coronary stents

4 Prosthetic valves

5 Artificial heart

Operations

1 Coronary artery bypass

2 Balloon angioplasty

3 Valve repair and replacement

4 Heart transplantation

5 Artificial heart operations

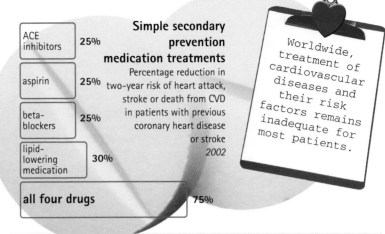

Simple secondary prevention medication treatments

Percentage reduction in two-year risk of heart attack, stroke or death from CVD in patients with previous coronary heart disease or stroke
2002

ACE inhibitors	25%
aspirin	25%
beta-blockers	25%
lipid-lowering medication	30%
all four drugs	75%

Worldwide, treatment of cardiovascular diseases and their risk factors remains inadequate for most patients.

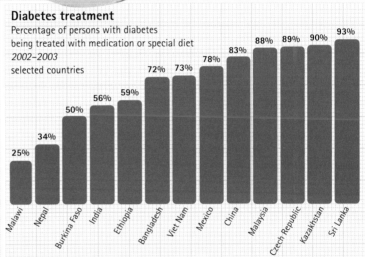

Diabetes treatment

Percentage of persons with diabetes being treated with medication or special diet
2002–2003
selected countries

- Malawi 25%
- Nepal 34%
- Burkina Faso 50%
- India 56%
- Ethiopia 59%
- Bangladesh 72%
- Viet Nam 73%
- Mexico 78%
- China 83%
- Malaysia 88%
- Czech Republic 89%
- Kazakhstan 90%
- Sri Lanka 93%

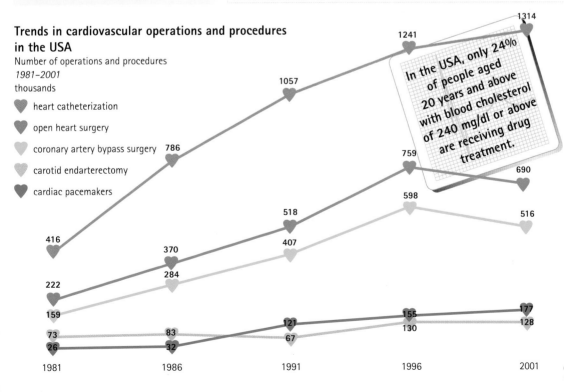

Trends in cardiovascular operations and procedures in the USA

Number of operations and procedures
1981–2001
thousands

- heart catheterization
- open heart surgery
- coronary artery bypass surgery
- carotid endarterectomy
- cardiac pacemakers

In the USA, only 24% of people aged 20 years and above with blood cholesterol of 240 mg/dl or above are receiving drug treatment.

heart catheterization: 416 (1981), 786 (1986), 1057 (1991), 1241 (1996), 1314 (2001)

coronary artery bypass surgery: 159 (1981), 284 (1986), 407 (1991), 598 (1996), 516 (2001)

open heart surgery: 222 (1981), 370 (1986), 518 (1991), 759 (1996), 690 (2001)

carotid endarterectomy: 73 (1981), 83 (1986), 121 (1991), 155 (1996), 177 (2001)

cardiac pacemakers: 26 (1981), 32 (1986), 67 (1991), 130 (1996), 128 (2001)

1981   1986   1991   1996   2001

71

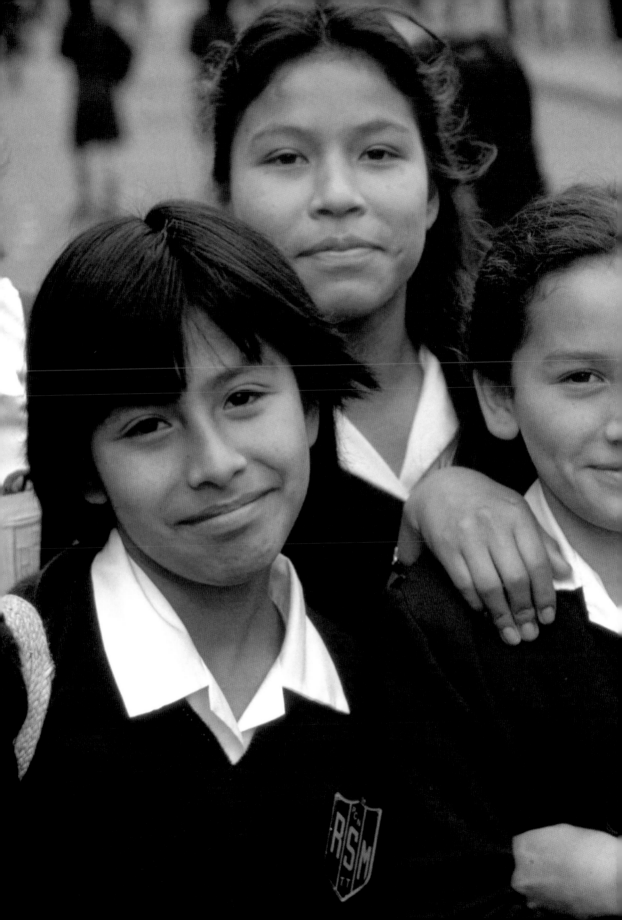

THE FUTURE AND THE PAST

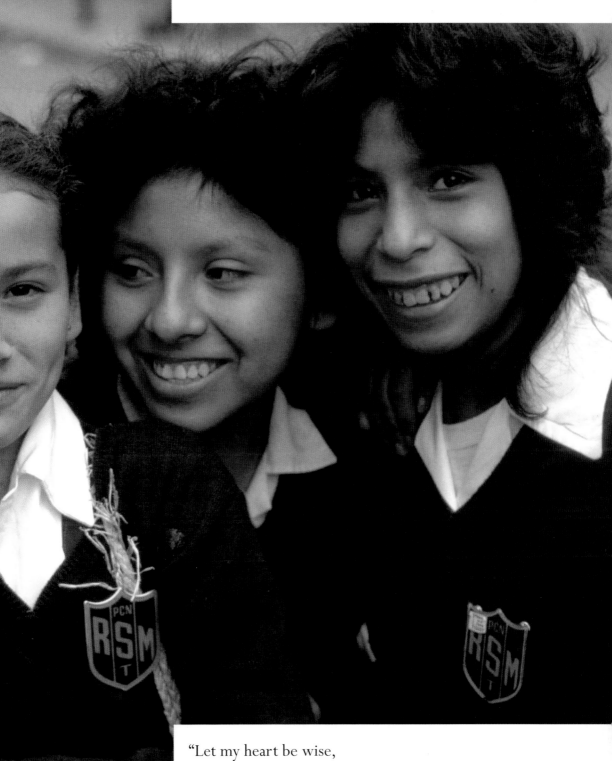

"Let my heart be wise,
It is the gods' best gift."

Euripides *Medea*, 431 BCE

The future

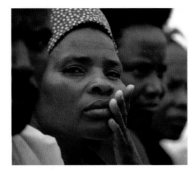

Unlike Einstein, we have to think of the future, and plan now, to reduce the numbers of deaths from coronary heart disease and stroke.

Predictions are by their nature speculative. Nevertheless, this much is certain: the global epidemic of cardiovascular disease is not only increasing, but also shifting from developed to developing nations.

Action can work. There are currently about 800 million people with high blood pressure worldwide. Studies now indicate that in North America, Western Europe, and the Asia-Pacific region, each 10 mmHg lowering of systolic blood pressure is associated with a decrease in risk of stroke of approximately one-third, in people aged 60 to 79 years. Globally, if diastolic blood pressure (DBP) can be reduced by 2%, and by 7% in those with DBP over 95 mmHg, a million deaths a year from coronary heart disease and stroke could be averted by 2020 in Asia alone.

No matter what advances there are in high-technology medicine, the fundamental message is that any major reduction in deaths and disability from CVD will come from prevention, not cure. This must involve robust reduction of risk factors.

"Unless current trends are halted or reversed, over a billion people will die from cardiovascular disease in the first half of the 21st century. The large majority will be in developing countries and much of the life years will be lost in middle age. This would be an enormous tragedy, given that research in the last half of the 20th century showed that cardiovascular disease was largely preventable."

Anthony Rodgers, Clinical Trials Research Unit, University of Auckland, New Zealand, 2004

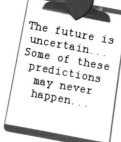

The future is uncertain... Some of these predictions may never happen...

DALYs	by 2010	by 2020	by 2030
CVD DALYs Annual number of DALYs	153 million	169 million	187 million
Burden of CVD Percentage of all DALYs	10.4%	11.0%	11.6%
CVD rankings globally	3rd: coronary heart disease 5th: stroke	3rd: coronary heart disease 4th: stroke	3rd: coronary heart disease 4th: stroke
CVD rankings in developing countries	4th: coronary heart disease 8th: stroke	3rd: coronary heart disease 6th: stroke	3rd: coronary heart disease 5th: stroke

DALYs Disability-adjusted life years combine years of potential life lost due to premature death with years of productive life lost due to disability.

DEATHS	by 2010	by 2020	by 2030
CVD deaths Annual number of deaths	18.1 million	20.5 million	24.2 million
CVD deaths Percentage of all deaths	30.8%	31.5%	32.5%
Coronary heart disease deaths Percentage of all male deaths	13.1%	14.3%	14.9%
Coronary heart disease deaths Percentage of all female deaths	13.6%	13.0%	13.1%
Stroke deaths Percentage of all male deaths	9.2%	9.8%	10.4%
Stroke deaths Percentage of all female deaths	11.5%	11.5%	11.8%
CVD deaths from cigarette smoking Annual number of deaths	1.9 million	2.6 million	

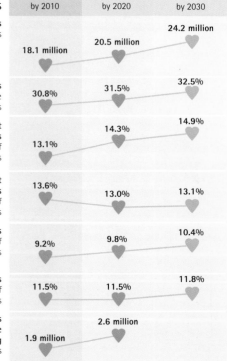

RISK FACTORS

RISK FACTORS	by 2010	by 2020	by 2030
Smokers — Number	1.3–1.4 billion	1.4–1.6 billion	1.4–1.8 billion
Diabetes — Number of people aged 20 years and above	221 million	300 million	366 million
Miscellaneous		Serious increases in LDL-cholesterol in many developing populations.	Short-term, long-term, and lifetime absolute risk of coronary heart disease and stroke routinely calculated by health care providers for everyone.

ECONOMIC COSTS

ECONOMIC COSTS	by 2010	by 2020	by 2030
Obesity-related complications — Percentage of health care spending in the USA, people aged 50 to 69 years	15%	20%	25%

ACTION

ACTION	by 2010	by 2020	by 2030
Research and development	New causal factors discovered for heart disease, including bacteria and viruses.	All newborn babies discharged home with CD-ROM containing their unique genomic maps, with summaries of CVD, of which they may be at increased risk. External glucose sensor will drive insulin pumps to deliver continuous microdoses of insulin. Vaccine produced to switch off nicotine receptors.	Bio-engineered tissues available for all heart and vascular structures.
UN Conventions and Goals	WHO Framework Convention on Tobacco Control (FCTC) ratified. WHO Global Strategy on Chronic Diseases, Diet and Physical Inactivity (2004).	Convention on Food ratified (covering content, labelling, taxation, advertising). Millennium Development Goals (2015): access to affordable essential drugs in developing countries provided, in cooperation with pharmaceutical companies.	Convention on universal access to essential preventive health care, and principles of equity in quality care delivery.

TREATMENT

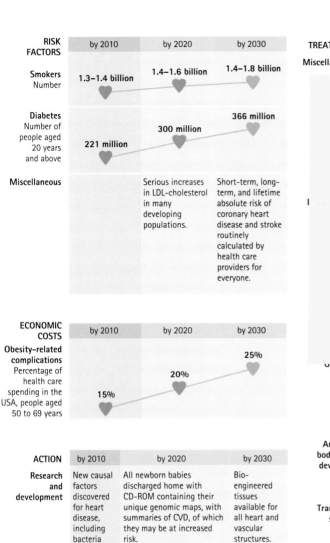

TREATMENT	by 2010	by 2020	by 2030
Miscellaneous	Full personal medical	Health systems driven by primary health care	Patients' knowledge of their
Genetics	CVD-modifying genes identified.	Genetic manipulation to prevent and treat CVD, including post-operative prevention of re-stenosis of arteries.	
Artificial body parts developed	Heart	Lungs	Brain add-ons Nerves to transplanted hearts
Transplant surgery		Xenotransplantation with pig hearts soars as rejection problem overcome.	Pig-napping of personal transgenic pigs a new crime.
High technology		Nano-surgeons, or sub-microscopic robots, will crawl through arteries, scraping away fatty deposits and repairing damaged or diseased parts. Angiogenesis, the growth of new blood vessels, may become an alternative to coronary bypass, angioplasty or clot-buster drugs.	Computerized "auto-doc" machine externally detects and treats illness by magnetic resonance therapy. Off-pump beating heart surgery predominates. Automated external defibrillators offered as routine electronic options in new homes for persons at high risk of sudden death.
Medication		Six-drug "polypill" will reduce CVD by more than 80% if taken by everyone aged 55 and older, and everyone with existing CVD.	Drugs developed to raise HDL-cholesterol (as effective as statins are today for lowering LDL-cholesterol).

Milestones in knowledge of heart and vascular disorders

Palaeolithic era *Spain* Oldest anatomical drawing in El Pindal cave of a mammoth with a dark smudge at the shoulder, which is thought to represent the heart.

2698–2598 BCE *China* Huang Ti, the Yellow Emperor, was thousands of years ahead of his time in writing in Nei Ching (Canon of Medicine): "The blood current flows continuously in a circle without a beginning or end and never stops" and "all the blood is under control of the heart". He also recorded the association between salt intake and a "hardened pulse".

1550 BCE *Egypt* Papyrus Ebers stated that after death the heart becomes the witness of the body's behaviour during life. To avoid incriminating testimony, the Egyptians buried the heart separately from the body.

600 BCE *Greece* Alcmaeon noted empty arteries in animals after death and inferred that arteries normally contained air.

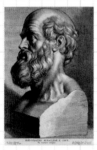

400 BCE *Greece* Hippocrates, the Father of Medicine (460–370 BCE), challenged the belief that illness was caused by the gods; he believed illness was caused by an imbalance of the four bodily humours: yellow bile, black bile, blood, and phlegm. He was also the first to recognize stroke.

310–250 BCE *Egypt* Erasistratus described the heart, veins, arteries and valves, but claimed that

arteries contained "pneuma" (air or spirit or soul), which was replaced each time a person breathed; when an artery was cut, blood rushed in as the pneuma escaped.

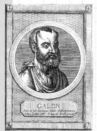

131–201 CE Graeco-Roman physician Claudius Galen, with knowledge gained from animals killed by Roman gladiators, described the heart and the movement of blood in the arteries, but claimed that the liver was the centre of the circulation and that the blood passed from the right to the left side of the heart.

980–1037 *Persia* Avicenna (Ibn Sina) stated that the heart is located centrally to all organs of the body, and that the left side of the heart was created as a store of spirit and soul.

1210–1288 *Syria* Ibn al-Nafis described the pulmonary and coronary circulation in *The Perfect Man*.

1452–1519 *Italy* Leonardo da Vinci incorrectly drew the liver as the centre of circulation. But he stated "vessels in the elderly through the thickening of the tunics, restrict the transit of the blood." This is one of the earliest descriptions of arteriosclerosis.

1509–1553 *Spain* Michael Servetus described the pulmonary circulation in his book *Christianismi Restitutio*.

1510–1559 *Padua, Italy* Matteo Realdo Colombo described the heart valves.

1525–1603 *Rome, Italy* Andrea Cesalpino noted that the circulation system is a closed system, and was the first in modern times to coin the term "blood circulation".

1553–1619 *Padua, Italy* Hieronymus Fabricius demonstrated valves in veins, which help to "prevent dilatation of veins".

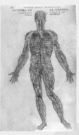

1555 *Padua, Italy* Andreas Vesalius (1514–1564) stated that the heart, and not the liver, was the centre of the circulation.

1559 *Italy* Riva di Trento discovered that there are two coronary arteries, each supplying blood to half of the heart.

1628 *England* William Harvey (1578–1657), a physician, published his thesis that the heart pumped blood around the body, in *De Motu Cordis*.

mid-1600s *Switzerland* Jacob Wepfer found that patients who died with "apoplexy" had bleeding in the brain. He also discovered that a blockage in one of the brain's blood vessels could cause apoplexy.

1706 *France* Anatomy professor Raymond de Vieussens first described the structure of the heart's chambers and vessels.

1712–1780 *England* John Fothergill both forecast the role of psychosocial factors and advised that a restricted diet "might greatly retard the progress" of coronary heart disease.

1677–1761 *England* Stephen Hales, an English clergyman and scientist, first measured blood pressure by inserting a brass tube into the artery of a horse. This was a scientific experiment, published in 1733, demonstrating that the heart exerts pressure in order to pump blood. The horse died.

1745–1827 *Italy* Alessandro Volta discovered that electric energy was produced by heart muscle contractions.

1749–1832 *England* Edward Jenner, better know for smallpox vaccine, made the essential link between angina pectoris and disease of the coronary arteries.

1752–1832 *Italy* Antonio Scarpa described arterial aneurysm.

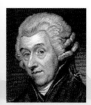

1772 *England* William Heberden (1710–1801) described angina pectoris: "they who are afflicted with it, are seized while they are walking (especially if it be uphill, and soon after eating) with a painful and most disagreeable sensation in the breast, which seems as if it would extinguish life if it were to increase or to continue; but the moment they stand still, all this uneasiness vanishes". He was also the first to write about hyperlipidaemia as a risk factor when he noticed that the serum of an obese patient who suddenly died was "thick like cream".

1775 *Scotland* John Hunter (1728–1793), a surgical pathologist, wrote "in a sudden and violent transport of anger, he fell down and expired immediately", illustrating the importance of emotion, stress and anger in precipitating coronary death. Hunter himself suffered from angina pectoris and died suddenly after a violent argument with a hospital colleague.

1785 *England* William Withering described the use of digitalis in coronary heart disease in his monograph *An Account of the Foxglove*. Foxglove had been used for centuries by American Indians.

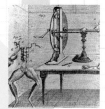

1791 *Italy* Luigi Galvani discovered that electrical stimulation of a frog's heart led to contraction of the cardiac muscle.

1799 *England* Caleb Hillier found something hard and gritty in the coronary arteries during an autopsy and "well remembered looking up to the ceiling, which was old and crumbling, conceiving that some plaster had fallen down". He discovered, however, that the vessels had hardened, and stated that "a principle cause of the syncope anginosa is to be looked for in disordered coronary arteries".

1815 *England* London surgeon Joseph Hodgson claimed inflammation was the underlying cause of atherosclerosis and it was not a natural degenerative part of the ageing process.

1815 *France* M.E. Chevreul named the fatty substance extracted from gallstones "cholesterol" from the Greek "khole" (bile) and "stereos" (solid).

1819 *France* Rene Theophile Laennec (1781–1826), invented the stethoscope. He rolled paper into a cylinder while examining a young woman with cardiac symptoms as he was reluctant to apply his ear to the chest.

1838 *France* Louis René Lecanu showed that cholesterol was present in human blood.

1841 *Austria* Carl Von Rokitansky championed the thrombogenic theory, proposing that deposits observed in the inner layer of the arterial wall derived primarily from fibrin and other blood elements rather than being the result of a purulent process. This theory came under attack from Rudolf Virchow.

1843 J. Vogel showed that cholesterol was present in atherosclerotic plaques.

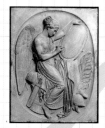

1844 *Denmark* First pathology report of plaque rupture in a coronary artery in Bertel Thorvaldsen, the celebrated neoclassical Danish artist and sculptor, who died of sudden cardiac death in the Royal Theatre in Copenhagen.

1850 Ventricular fibrillation first described.

1850s Ophthalmoscope invented, allowing direct visualization of arteries at the back of the eye.

1852 *England* Fatty material in the coronary arteries described by Sir Richard Quain, which he attributed to nutrition. He linked the fatty heart to "languid and feeble circulation, a sense of uneasiness and oppression in the chest, embarrassment and distress in breathing, coma, syncope, angina pectoris, sudden death…"

1856–1967

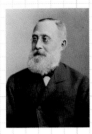

1856 *Germany* Rudolf Virchow, a Pole, believed that disease occurred at cellular level, and also described cerebral emboli causing stroke. Virchow also emphasized the societal causes of disease as "disturbances of human culture".

1867 *England* Lauder Brunton, pharmacologist, discovered that amyl nitrite relieved angina.

1872 *France* Gabriel Lippmann invented the capillary electrometer, the precursor of the electrocardiograph.

1893 *Holland* Willem Einthoven (1860–1927) introduced the term electrocardiogram or ECG/EKG; distinguished five deflections – PQRST (1895); constructed the first electrocardiograph in 1901, which weighed 270 kg, occupied two rooms and required five people to operate it; transmitted the first ECG from hospital to his laboratory 1.5 km away via telephone cable (in 1905); published the first normal and abnormal ECGs (1906) and won the Nobel Prize (1924).

1895 *Germany* Physicist Wilhem Konrad Roentgen (1845–1923) discovered X-rays, which are still used to visualize the heart.

1896 *Italy* Scipione Riva-Rocci invented the sphygmomanometer to measure blood pressure.

1897 The introduction of modern aspirin. In one of life's little ironies, Bayer's first aspirin advertisements said that the drug did "not affect the heart".

1906 *Germany* M. Cremer, first oesophageal ECG by a professional sword swallower. First fetal ECG from the abdominal surface of a pregnant woman.

1907 *England* First case report of atrial fibrillation by Arthur Cushny, professor of pharmacology at University College, London.

1912 James B. Herrick described heart disease resulting from hardening of the arteries.

1912 First human cardiac catheterization (no X-ray visualization) by Frizt Bleichroeder, E. Unger and W. Loeb.

1915 *USA* Establishment of organization in New York City, which became the American Heart Association.

1920 *USA* First ECG of acute myocardial infarction by Harold Pardee.

1923 *USA* First operative widening of scarred cardiac valve by E. Cutler and S.A. Levine.

1925 *United Kingdom* Widening of narrowed mitral valve by Souter, who stretched the valve ring with his fingers.

1928 *United Kingdom* Sir Alexander Fleming discovered penicillin, which is used to treat rheumatic fever.

1928 "Apoplexy" divided into categories based on the cause of the blood vessel problem, and replaced by the term "cerebral vascular accident (CVA)".

1929 *Germany* First documented right heart catheterization in human by Werner Forssmann using radiographic techniques.

1931 *USA* First description of the use of exercise to provoke attacks of angina pectoris by Charles Wolferth and Francis Wood.

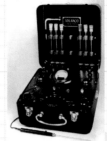

1931 *USA* First artificial cardiac pacemaker, which stimulated the heart by transthoracic needle, developed by Dr Albert Hyman.

1937 *USA* First prototype heart-lung machine built by physician John Heysham Gibbon, and tested on animals. He performed the first human open heart operation in 1953 using the machine.

1938 *USA* First human heart surgery, first surgical correction of a congenital heart defect: closure of patent ductus arteriosus performed by surgeon Robert E. Gross.

1944 *China* First repair of patent ductus arteriosus in China.

1944 *USA* First operation on "blue baby" (Fallot's tetralogy) at Johns Hopkins.

1944 *USA/Sweden* First repair of coarctation of aorta by Crafoord and Grosse.

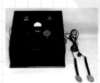

1947 *USA* First defibrillation of human heart during cardiac surgery, by Claude Beck in Cleveland.

1948 *USA* "Blind finger" closed heart surgery for mitral stenosis reintroduced by Dr Dwight Harken and Dr Charles Bailey.

1948 *USA* California physician Lawrence Craven noticed that 400 of his male patients who took aspirin for two years had no heart attacks. By 1956, he had chronicled the health of 8000 patients taking aspirin and found no heart attacks in the group.

1948 *USA* Start of the Framingham Heart Study where, for the first time, a large cohort of healthy men and women were studied prospectively.

1949 *USA* Portable Holter Monitor invented by Norman Jeff Holter to record ambulatory ECG.

1950 The International Society of Cardiology established, later joined with International Cardiology Federation and renamed World Heart Federation.

1950 *Canada* First pacemaker invented by John Hopps.

1952 *USA* First prosthetic valve implanted in aorta by surgeon Charles Hufnagel.

1952 *USA* First successful human open heart surgery under hypothermia by Walton Lillehei and John Lewis, who implanted the first synthetic valve in a five-year-old girl who had been born with an atrioseptal defect (hole in her heart).

1952 *USA* External cardiac pacemaker designed by Paul Zoll.

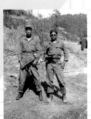

1953 *USA* First demonstrated coronary artery disease among young US soldiers killed in action in Korea (later observed in the casualties of the Viet Nam War too) by William F. Enos, Robert H. Holmes and James Beyer.

1954 *United Kingdom* First carotid endarterectomy by Eastcott, Pickering and Rob.

1954 *India* Called on WHO to address the coming epidemic of cardiovascular disease in developing countries.

1955 *United Kingdom* First reported mitral valve replacement by Judson Chesterman.

1950s Minimization of bias for the reliable assessment of cardiovascular treatments by introduction of randomization into clinical trials (at instigation of Sir Austin Bradford Hill).

1956 *USA* First report of the successful ending of ventricular fibrillation in humans by externally applied countershock published by Dr Paul Zoll.

1957 First battery-powered external pacemaker.

1958 *USA* Seymour Furman inserted a pacemaker in a patient who lived for 96 days.

1958 *Sweden* Internal long-term cardiac pacing by Åke Senning.

1958 Start of development of a selective coronary angiography procedure by Mason Sones.

1959 WHO established Cardiovascular Diseases programme.

1960s High blood pressure identified as a treatable risk factor for stroke.

1960 *USA* First Coronary Care Unit in Bethany, Kansas.

1960 *Framingham, USA* Cigarette smoking found to increase the risk of heart disease.

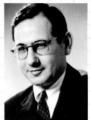

1960 *USA* First replacement of heart valve with Starr-Edwards mechanical valve, developed by Albert Starr (*left*) and Lowell Edwards.

1961 *USA* Framingham Heart Study investigators coined the term "risk factors" for the development of coronary heart disease. High cholesterol level, blood pressure, and electrocardiogram abnormalities found to increase the risk of coronary heart disease.

1961 *USA* First use of external cardiac massage to restart a heart by J.R. Jude.

1961 *USA* First direct current defibrillation with external paddles by Bernard Lown and Barough Berkowitz.

1960s First human implant of totally implantable pacemaker.

1964 *USA* First transluminal angioplasty performed on a narrowed artery in the leg by Charles T. Dotter.

1965 *USA* Michael DeBakey and Adrian Kantrowitz implanted mechanical devices to help a diseased heart.

1967 *South Africa* First whole heart transplant from one person to another by Dr Christiaan Barnard.

1967 *USA* Saphenous vein coronary bypass graft by Dr Rene Favaloro.

1967 *Framingham, USA* Physical inactivity and obesity found to increase the risk of heart disease.

1969 *USA* First use of artificial heart in human by Denton Cooley.

1972 *USA* The Stanford Three Community Study started (later becoming The Stanford Five-City Project); this showed a 23% reduction in coronary heart disease risk caused by community-based interventions that change lifestyle-related risk factors such as physical activity, dietary habits and tobacco use.

1972 *Finland* North Karelia Project began, aimed at preventing cardiovascular disease among residents. Cardiovascular mortality rates for men, aged between 35 and 64 years, decreased by 57% from 1970 to 1992.

1974 *Framingham, USA* Diabetes linked to cardiovascular disease.

1970s Aspirin recognized as preventing heart attacks and stroke.

1970s Development of computerized tomography (CT) to aid early diagnosis of stroke.

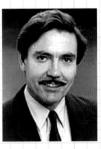

1977 *Switzerland* First coronary PTCA (percutaneous transluminal coronary angioplasty); Andreas Gruentzig inserted a balloon-tipped catheter into a coronary artery and inflated the balloon, and thus successfully opened a blockage and restored blood flow.

1977 *Italy* The Martignacco Project community prevention trial resulted in reduction of coronary heart disease through community-based interventions that change lifestyle-related risk factors such as physical activity, dietary habits and tobacco use.

1977 *Framingham, USA* Effects described of triglycerides and LDL- and HDL- cholesterol on heart disease.

1978 *Framingham, USA* Psychosocial factors found to affect heart disease.

1978 *Australia* North Coast Healthy Lifestyle Programme showed significant reduction in smoking.

1978 *Switzerland* Swiss National Research Programme community prevention trial resulted in reduction of smoking, blood pressure and obesity.

1978 Atrial fibrillation (irregular heart beat) found to increase the risk of stroke.

1979 *South Africa* Coronary Risk Factor Study community prevention trial resulted in reduction of smoking, blood pressure and composite coronary heart disease risks.

1979 *Germany* First use by Peter Rentrop of intracoronary streptokinase, a clot-dissolving drug to stop a heart attack in progress.

1981 *Framingham, USA* Filter cigarettes found to carry as much risk for coronary heart disease as unfiltered cigarettes.

1981 *USA* Report on relationship between diet and heart disease.

1982 *USA* First permanent artificial heart, designed by Robert Jarvik, and implanted by Willem DeVries, in a 61-year-old man.

1983 *USA* List of 246 coronary risk factors published by Hopkins and Williams (list now much longer).

1980s Minimization of random error for the reliable assessment of cardiovascular treatments by introduction of large-scale "mega-trials" (at instigation of Sir Richard Peto).

1986 *France* First coronary stent implanted by Jacques Puel and Ulrich Sigwart.

1987 *Japan* M. Okada used a laser to burn channels in the heart muscle to help revascularize the heart in patients with coronary heart disease.

1987 *Framingham, USA* High blood cholesterol levels found to correlate directly with risk of death in young men.

1988 *Framingham, USA* High levels of HDL-cholesterol found to reduce risk of death.

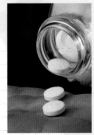

1988 ISIS-2 trial shows emergency treatment for heart attacks with aspirin and fibrinolytic "clot-busting" drugs saves lives.

1988 *Framingham, USA* Isolated systolic hypertension found to increase risk of heart disease.

1988 *Framingham, USA* Cigarette smoking found to increase risk of stroke.

1990 Randomized trials showed that lowering blood pressure lowers the risk of stroke.

1990 *United Kingdom* Meta-analysis of trials by Clinical Trial Service Unit (CTSU) in Oxford showed that lowering blood pressure lowers the risk of coronary disease.

1991 *China* Tianjin CVD Intervention Programme community prevention trial led to the creation of non-smoking environments and increased sales of low-sodium seasonings.

1992 *Canada* The Victoria Declaration on Heart Health affirmed that CVD is largely preventable, that there is the scientific knowledge to eliminate most CVD, and that the public health infrastructure and capacity to address prevention were lacking.

1990s *USA* Hostility (including traits such as anger, cynicism, and mistrust), a major component of type A behaviour, shown to be associated with an increased risk of heart attack and other cardiac complications in healthy persons and patients with coronary heart disease.

1992 *China* First heart-lung transplant in China.

mid-1990s *Scandinavia, United Kingdom, USA* Remarkable improvement in survival of coronary heart disease patients treated with statins.

1995 *Spain* The Catalonia Declaration: Investing in Heart Health, and its follow-up convention in 1997, emphasized the importance of investments in heart health and provided examples of many successful CVD prevention programmes worldwide.

1998 *USA* Hypertension gene in men identified.

1998 New advances: gene therapy grows new blood vessels to the heart; strong confirmation that "superaspirin"

IIb/IIIa receptor blocker drugs prevent blood clots; the importance of inflammation in cardiovascular disease recognized; study on the deadly effects of smoking fewer than 10 cigarettes per day.

1998 *Singapore* The Singapore Declaration: Forging the Will for Heart Health in the Next Millennium.

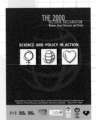

2000 *Canada* The Victoria Declaration on Women, Heart Disease and Stroke addressed the importance of science and policy in action and the need to tackle gender disparities in health. It called upon all stakeholders to join forces and take appropriate action to control the cardiovascular disease epidemic.

2000 First World Heart Day, which has become a global annual event.

2000 The entire human genome is mapped.

2000 WHO 53rd World Health Assembly endorsed Global strategy for noncommunicable disease (NCD) prevention and control, which outlines major objectives for monitoring, preventing and managing NCDs with special emphasis on major NCDs with common risk factors and determinants – cardiovascular disease, cancer, diabetes and chronic respiratory disease.

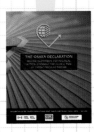

2001 *Japan* The Osaka Declaration: Health, Economics and Political Action: Stemming the Global Tide of

Cardiovascular Disease emphasized the global nature of the CVD burden and highlighted the need to address economic and political factors in order to tackle CVD.

2002 *United Kingdom* The Heart Protection Study showed that statins could benefit people with diabetes and those with cholesterol levels previously considered low.

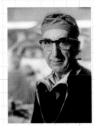

2002 *USA* NASA's Commercial Invention of the Year Award given for the DeBakey Ventricular Assist Device, based on space shuttle technology, and developed by Michael DeBakey *(above)* and NASA engineer David Saucier. The pump, used to treat heart failure, was one-tenth the size of previous heart-assist devices, and was first used in a patient in 2000.

2003 *Switzerland* WHO Framework Convention on Tobacco Control adopted at the 56th World Health Assembly.

2003 *Switzerland* The World Health Report: "Shaping the Future" highlighted CVD as the first of three growing threats that make up the "neglected global epidemics". The report called for action at the national and global levels to prevent and control CVD.

2004 *Switzerland* WHO Global Strategy on Diet, Physical Activity and Health endorsed by World Health Assembly.

2004 *Italy* Milan Declaration on Heart Health: Positioning Technology to serve Global Heart Health.

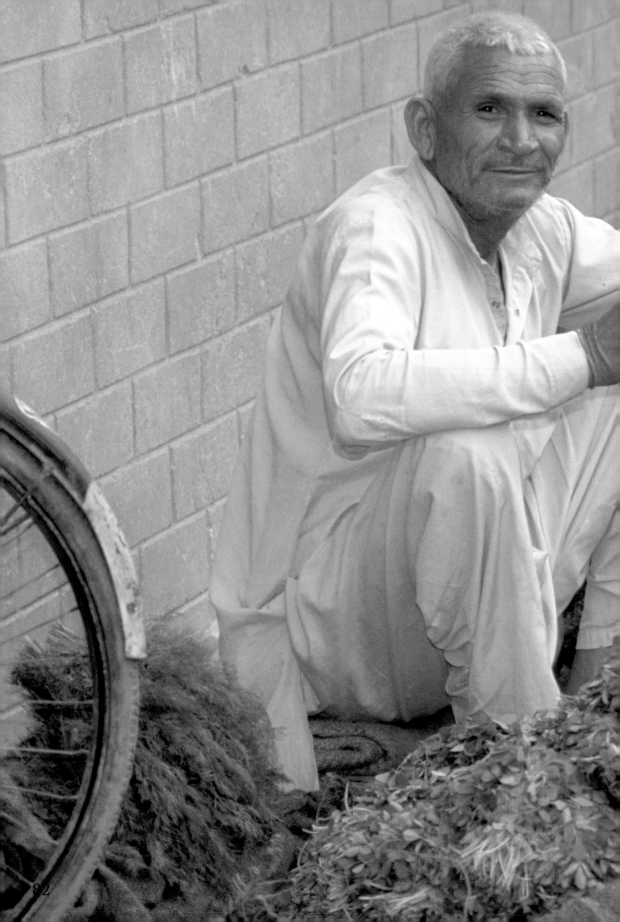

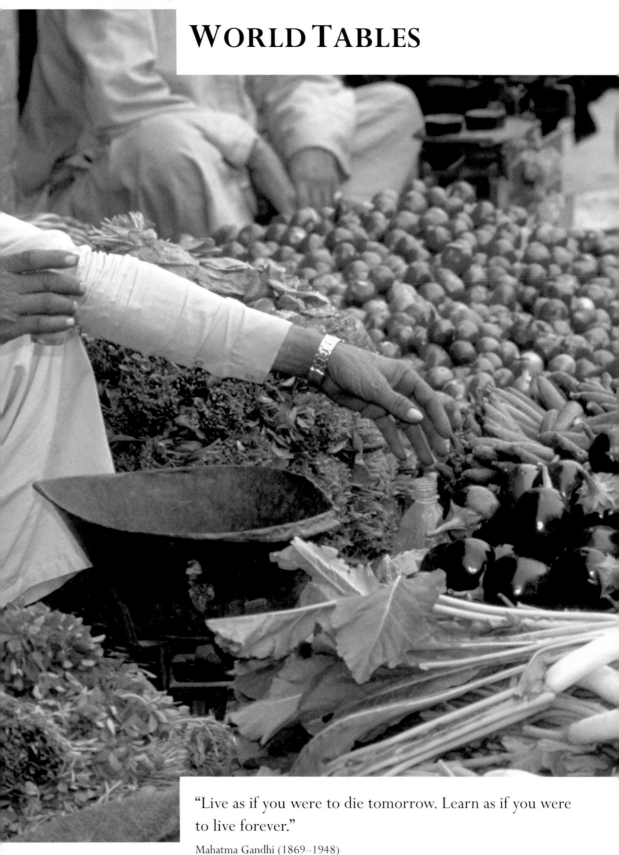

PART 6

WORLD TABLES

"Live as if you were to die tomorrow. Learn as if you were to live forever."

Mahatma Gandhi (1869–1948)

World Data Table

Country	1 Population Thousands 2002	2 Heart disease Disability DALYS lost per 1000 population 2002	2 Heart disease Mortality Number of deaths 2002	3 Stroke Disability DALYS lost per 1000 population 2003 or latest available data	3 Stroke Mortality Number of deaths 2002	4 Rheumatic heart disease Number of deaths 2002
Afghanistan	22 930	36	33 157	13	11 532	1 938
Albania	3 141	13	3 989	13	4 169	42
Algeria	31 266	7	14 948	8	16 223	756
Andorra	69	3	67	3	52	3
Angola	13 184	13	7 130	15	7 640	615
Antigua and Barbuda	73	6	52	13	92	0
Argentina	37 981	6	34 292	6	22 668	234
Armenia	3 072	20	8 515	10	4 212	151
Australia	19 544	5	25 474	3	11 730	243
Austria	8 111	6	15 418	4	7 559	185
Azerbaijan	8 297	28	22 302	9	6 540	184
Bahamas	310	5	154	6	155	1
Bahrain	709	8	283	3	84	6
Bangladesh	143 809	18	130 006	9	64 515	10 253
Barbados	269	6	286	7	270	2
Belarus	9 940	28	59 719	14	22 892	550
Belgium	10 296	5	14 985	4	9 234	68
Belize	251	8	153	7	111	1
Benin	6 558	10	3 017	12	3 279	236
Bhutan	2 190	20	2 672	10	1 370	195
Bolivia	8 645	6	3 948	7	3 138	70
Bosnia and Herzegovina	4 126	10	5 590	13	6 508	21
Botswana	1 770	8	697	8	670	15
Brazil	176 257	9	139 601	11	129 172	3 055
Brunei Darussalam	350	5	92	6	90	7
Bulgaria	7 965	14	26 243	13	20 882	232
Burkina Faso	12 624	11	5 877	13	6 604	466
Burundi	6 602	10	3 084	12	3 492	82
Cambodia	13 810	13	7 635	11	5 963	614
Cameroon	15 729	10	9 443	12	10 198	621
Canada	31 271	5	43 246	3	15 621	422
Cape Verde	454	6	202	9	266	4
Central African Rep.	3 819	10	2 513	12	2 727	51
Chad	8 348	10	4 385	12	4 747	300
Chile	15 613	4	9 075	5	8 142	315
China	1 294 867	4	702 925	12	1 652 885	97 245
Colombia	43 526	8	31 289	6	17 745	380
Comoros	747	8	282	10	310	23
Congo	3 633	9	1 577	10	1 718	39
Congo, Dem. Rep.	51 201	11	24 217	13	26 439	1 930
Cook Islands	18	10	11	12	11	0
Costa Rica	4 094	6	2 937	3	1 194	45
Côte d'Ivoire	16 365	11	9 257	12	9 530	233
Croatia	4 439	10	11 653	11	8 653	152
Cuba	11 271	8	16 275	5	7 684	196
Cyprus	796	7	1 358	3	795	1
Czech Republic	10 246	11	25 899	7	15 663	286
Denmark	5 351	5	10 013	4	4 871	17

5 Smoking prevalence		6 Diabetes	7 Research	8 Policies and legislation	Country
Percentage of people 18 years and above who smoke *2003 or latest available data*		Percentage of people aged 20 years and above with diabetes *2000*	Number of publications on cardiovascular disease *1991–2001*	Legal status of smoking in government buildings *2004 or latest available data*	
men	women				
–	–	4.7%	–	unknown	Afghanistan
46.2%	22.8%	4.5%	–	not regulated	Albania
40.2%	11.5%	2.6%	1	unknown	Algeria
49.6%	35.9%	8.8%	–	banned	Andorra
–	–	0.9%	–	not regulated	Angola
–	–	7.3%	–	unknown	Antigua and Barbuda
32.0%	18.9%	6.1%	110	not regulated	Argentina
67.4%	4.1%	4.7%	1	not regulated	Armenia
30.7%	23.1%	6.8%	710	restricted	Australia
37.4%	26.3%	3.8%	320	restricted	Austria
32.0%	1.7%	6.8%	1	banned	Azerbaijan
–	–	6.2%	–	unknown	Bahamas
29.5%	16.0%	9.1%	4	unknown	Bahrain
63.0%	34.5%	4.6%	3	restricted	Bangladesh
19.8%	3.0%	5.8%	1	banned	Barbados
63.6%	22.0%	9.9%	3	restricted	Belarus
33.2%	22.9%	4.0%	345	restricted	Belgium
–	–	4.2%	–	restricted	Belize
–	5.4%	3.3%	1	unknown	Benin
–	–	3.5%	–	unknown	Bhutan
36.7%	19.2%	4.9%	–	restricted	Bolivia
54.6%	31.5%	3.8%	–	banned	Bosnia and Herzegovina
–	–	3.6%	–	restricted	Botswana
29.4%	18.4%	4.3%	307	banned	Brazil
–	–	9.4%	–	banned	Brunei Darussalam
47.3%	28.2%	7.7%	18	banned	Bulgaria
25.6%	13.2%	2.7%	2	not regulated	Burkina Faso
–	–	1.0%	–	not regulated	Burundi
–	6.5%	1.9%	–	restricted	Cambodia
20.7%	2.4%	1.0%	4	restricted	Cameroon
30.0%	26.6%	8.8%	1 237	restricted	Canada
–	–	3.4%	–	restricted	Cape Verde
–	–	1.0%	–	not regulated	Central African Rep.
19.7%	3.1%	2.8%	–	not regulated	Chad
44.1%	36.6%	5.2%	53	restricted	Chile
58.9%	3.6%	2.4%	472	restricted	China
–	–	3.6%	11	unknown	Colombia
30.5%	18.4%	1.4%	–	unknown	Comoros
20.8%	3.9%	1.1%	2	restricted	Congo
–	–	1.4%	–	unknown	Congo, Dem. Rep.
–	–	6.3%	–	not regulated	Cook Islands
24.3%	10.0%	3.3%	2	restricted	Costa Rica
21.0%	4.0%	3.6%	–	restricted	Côte d'Ivoire
41.4%	27.4%	4.4%	41	banned	Croatia
48.8%	28.5%	6.0%	15	restricted	Cuba
–	–	9.2%	–	restricted	Cyprus
42.6%	26.2%	4.3%	78	banned	Czech Republic
40.3%	36.9%	3.8%	308	restricted	Denmark

World Data Table

Country	1 Population Thousands 2002	2 Heart disease Disability DALYS lost per 1000 population 2002	Mortality Number of deaths 2002	3 Stroke Disability DALYS lost per 1000 population 2003 or latest available data	Mortality Number of deaths 2002	4 Rheumatic heart disease Number of deaths 2002
Djibouti	693	21	727	7	248	27
Dominica	78	3	30	4	30	0
Dominican Republic	8 616	11	7 271	9	4 833	54
Ecuador	12 810	5	5 826	5	4 374	117
Egypt	70 507	21	103 829	8	35 054	3 398
El Salvador	6 415	10	5 328	4	1 684	39
Equatorial Guinea	481	11	313	12	333	18
Eritrea	3 991	9	1 326	10	1 474	42
Estonia	1 338	16	6 235	9	2 964	65
Ethiopia	68 961	10	32 477	11	35 329	2 482
Fiji	831	18	783	17	685	21
Finland	5 197	7	12 488	4	4 875	77
France	59 850	3	46 132	3	37 750	1 136
Gabon	1 306	11	1 001	11	951	57
Gambia	1 388	10	789	11	837	48
Georgia	5 177	23	26 035	17	15 680	59
Germany	82 414	6	172 717	4	79 326	2 241
Ghana	20 471	9	10 471	11	11 337	705
Greece	10 970	7	16 825	6	22 694	10
Grenada	80	9	85	13	91	1
Guatemala	12 036	4	2 796	4	2 232	14
Guinea	8 359	11	4 137	12	4 415	289
Guinea-Bissau	1 449	11	783	13	844	52
Guyana	764	12	791	18	880	8
Haiti	8 218	5	2 469	16	6 764	62
Honduras	6 781	10	4 544	8	2 786	79
Hungary	9 923	13	29 502	8	17 148	354
Iceland	287	5	416	3	189	3
India	1 049 549	20	1 531 534	10	771 067	103 913
Indonesia	217 131	14	220 372	8	123 684	11 660
Iran, Isl. Rep.	68 070	17	81 983	8	31 768	1 138
Iraq	24 510	19	22 036	8	8 291	695
Ireland	3 911	8	6 527	4	2 650	51
Israel	6 304	4	5 705	3	2 233	170
Italy	57 482	4	92 928	4	69 075	1 790
Jamaica	2 627	5	1 877	11	3 559	59
Japan	127 478	3	90 196	5	134 952	2 585
Jordan	5 329	13	3 788	6	1 428	127
Kazakhstan	15 469	28	51 948	17	26 874	919
Kenya	31 540	9	13 661	10	14 843	360
Kiribati	87	1	7	18	81	0
Korea, Dem. People's Rep. of	22 541	13	26 953	8	14 337	1 317
Korea, Republic of	47 430	3	15 811	9	46 151	202
Kuwait	2 443	10	940	3	213	7
Kyrgyzstan	5 067	22	10 850	22	8 366	351
Lao People's Dem. Rep.	5 529	19	5 539	12	3 620	484
Latvia	2 329	17	9 928	12	7 278	109
Lebanon	3 596	17	5 471	7	2 072	119

5 Smoking prevalence Percentage of people 18 years and above who smoke 2003 or latest available data		6 Diabetes Percentage of people aged 20 years and above with diabetes 2000	7 Research Number of publications on cardiovascular disease 1991–2001	8 Policies and legislation Legal status of smoking in government buildings 2004 or latest available data	Country
men	women				
–	–	2.5%	–	unknown	Djibouti
–	–	6.2%	–	unknown	Dominica
22.1%	16.2%	5.2%	–	restricted	Dominican Republic
31.9%	7.4%	4.8%	3	banned	Ecuador
47.9%	1.8%	7.2%	20	restricted	Egypt
–	–	3.0%	–	unknown	El Salvador
–	–	3.8%	–	unknown	Equatorial Guinea
–	–	2.8%	4	not regulated	Eritrea
57.1%	28.8%	4.4%	7	banned	Estonia
9.7%	0.8%	2.8%	4	not regulated	Ethiopia
47.3%	14.0%	8.3%	1	not regulated	Fiji
31.6%	22.3%	3.9%	331	banned	Finland
42.6%	33.9%	3.9%	1 407	restricted	France
–	–	1.2%	–	not regulated	Gabon
43.4%	6.2%	3.3%	4	restricted	Gambia
61.4%	6.3%	5.3%	159	not regulated	Georgia
39.0%	30.9%	4.1%	2 276	restricted	Germany
14.2%	1.9%	3.3%	1	restricted	Ghana
53.5%	33.6%	10.3%	245	restricted	Greece
–	–	7.3%	–	unknown	Grenada
24.5%	3.7%	2.7%	–	restricted	Guatemala
–	–	0.9%	3	banned	Guinea
–	–	3.1%	–	not regulated	Guinea-Bissau
–	–	4.2%	–	unknown	Guyana
25.2%	5.4%	4.1%	–	unknown	Haiti
–	–	2.7%	–	unknown	Honduras
47.2%	27.7%	4.4%	103	banned	Hungary
26.5%	27.1%	3.2%	9	banned	Iceland
34.6%	3.4%	5.5%	294	banned	India
59.8%	5.3%	6.7%	4	restricted	Indonesia
33.4%	3.5%	6.0%	–	banned	Iran, Isl. Rep.
–	–	6.1%	1	unknown	Iraq
33.8%	26.5%	3.2%	142	restricted	Ireland
35.8%	19.7%	6.7%	634	banned	Israel
37.9%	29.7%	9.2%	1 976	banned	Italy
56.1%	21.2%	5.4%	23	not regulated	Jamaica
52.5%	12.4%	6.7%	3 769	restricted	Japan
66.8%	5.3%	8.1%	6	banned	Jordan
57.5%	6.4%	4.4%	–	restricted	Kazakhstan
66.3%	27.3%	1.4%	3	not regulated	Kenya
–	–	8.6%	–	not regulated	Kiribati
–	–	2.5%	–	unknown	Korea, Dem. People's Rep. of
69.5%	5.1%	5.6%	19	restricted	Korea, Republic of
35.7%	2.7%	9.8%	17	restricted	Kuwait
64.1%	41.4%	3.6%	–	not regulated	Kyrgyzstan
68.9%	16.1%	1.8%	–	restricted	Lao People's Dem. Rep.
64.5%	29.2%	4.5%	1	restricted	Latvia
60.7%	46.9%	7.0%	65	restricted	Lebanon

World Data Table

Country	1 Population Thousands 2002	2 Heart disease		3 Stroke		4 Rheumatic heart disease
		Disability DALYS lost per 1000 population 2002	Mortality Number of deaths 2002	Disability DALYS lost per 1000 population 2003 or latest available data	Mortality Number of deaths 2002	Number of deaths 2002
Lesotho	1 800	9	1 200	11	1 299	24
Liberia	3 239	12	1 442	14	1 559	130
Libyan Arab Jamahiriya	5 445	15	5 309	6	1 762	130
Lithuania	3 465	16	14 662	7	5 089	186
Luxembourg	447	4	455	5	390	0
Macedonia, Former Yugos. Rep. of	2 046	9	2 544	13	3 772	41
Madagascar	16 916	10	8 327	11	9 020	609
Malawi	11 871	10	6 773	11	7 249	106
Malaysia	23 965	8	13 445	7	10 169	464
Maldives	309	17	282	10	152	16
Mali	12 623	11	5 406	13	5 946	478
Malta	393	9	865	4	338	6
Marshall Islands	52	20	57	20	54	2
Mauritania	2 807	11	1 640	13	1 756	111
Mauritius	1 210	18	2 034	11	1 235	5
Mexico	101 965	6	51 454	4	26 478	1 093
Micronesia, Federated States of	108	12	64	14	69	2
Moldova, Republic of	4 270	23	18 559	15	7 848	264
Monaco	34	3	27	3	22	1
Mongolia	2 559	8	1 153	25	2 515	145
Morocco	30 072	14	29 934	5	10 607	808
Mozambique	18 537	8	7 969	10	8 896	246
Myanmar	48 852	17	58 478	11	33 406	3 746
Namibia	1 961	8	996	10	1 108	25
Nauru	13	22	17	10	7	0
Nepal	24 609	18	23 314	10	11 961	1 648
Netherlands	16 067	5	19 045	4	12 459	16
New Zealand	3 846	7	6 141	4	2 699	139
Nicaragua	5 335	8	2 680	7	1 768	70
Niger	11 544	11	4 423	13	4 831	439
Nigeria	120 911	11	64 778	12	69 932	4 795
Niue	2	10	1	12	1	0
Norway	4 514	5	8 886	3	4 817	103
Oman	2 768	17	1 765	4	375	12
Pakistan	149 911	18	154 338	9	78 512	11 604
Palau	20	14	17	14	16	0
Panama	3 064	5	1 628	5	1 489	30
Papua New Guinea	5 586	18	3 994	10	1 960	351
Paraguay	5 740	7	2 606	10	2 881	36
Peru	26 767	4	10 615	4	8 084	157
Philippines	78 580	10	45 378	7	24 368	2 812
Poland	38 622	10	77 151	7	43 032	1 277
Portugal	10 049	5	10 927	9	20 069	189
Qatar	601	9	238	4	75	4
Romania	22 387	13	60 718	13	52 272	566
Russian Federation	144 082	27	674 881	19	517 424	8 126
Rwanda	8 272	10	3 493	12	3 811	101
Saint Kitts and Nevis	42	10	46	19	84	0

5 Smoking prevalence Percentage of people 18 years and above who smoke 2003 or latest available data		6 Diabetes Percentage of people aged 20 years and above with diabetes 2000	7 Research Number of publications on cardiovascular disease 1991–2001	8 Policies and legislation Legal status of smoking in government buildings 2004 or latest available data	Country
men	women				
–	–	3.1%	–	unknown	Lesotho
–	–	3.1%	–	unknown	Liberia
–	–	3.1%	–	banned	Libyan Arab Jamahiriya
46.4%	15.9%	4.2%	5	restricted	Lithuania
41.4%	30.2%	3.6%	3	restricted	Luxembourg
–	–	3.8%	5	banned	Macedonia, Former Yugos. Rep. of
–	–	1.4%	2	not regulated	Madagascar
31.0%	7.4%	1.1%	1	not regulated	Malawi
52.4%	3.0%	7.6%	16	banned	Malaysia
–	–	5.0%	–	banned	Maldives
26.9%	4.7%	2.9%	–	restricted	Mali
–	–	13.9%	5	not regulated	Malta
–	–	8.6%	9	banned	Marshall Islands
25.0%	4.3%	2.8%	–	not regulated	Mauritania
54.7%	3.1%	14.6%	2	restricted	Mauritius
36.5%	14.3%	3.9%	201	restricted	Mexico
–	–	8.6%	–	not regulated	Micronesia, Federated States of
–	–	5.9%	–	restricted	Moldova, Republic of
–	–	8.8%	7	unknown	Monaco
46.2%	7.3%	2.5%	1	restricted	Mongolia
32.6%	0.6%	2.6%	7	restricted	Morocco
–	–	1.6%	1	unknown	Mozambique
55.5%	12.2%	2.0%	–	unknown	Myanmar
33.8%	16.1%	3.1%	–	not regulated	Namibia
56.8%	64.7%	27.8%	–	banned	Nauru
61.5%	34.6%	3.9%	3	banned	Nepal
38.3%	32.8%	3.5%	917	restricted	Netherlands
28.1%	28.7%	6.7%	131	restricted	New Zealand
–	–	2.9%	–	restricted	Nicaragua
–	–	2.5%	–	unknown	Niger
16.3%	3.6%	3.4%	18	banned	Nigeria
36.8%	14.0%	6.3%	–	restricted	Niue
40.3%	39.0%	3.9%	185	restricted	Norway
23.6%	2.9%	9.9%	19	unknown	Oman
30.3%	3.8%	7.7%	12	banned	Pakistan
50.9%	22.6%	8.6%	–	banned	Palau
35.1%	17.7%	3.5%	1	unknown	Panama
48.9%	–	6.5%	3	banned	Papua New Guinea
45.8%	15.6%	3.7%	1	restricted	Paraguay
–	–	5.2%	3	restricted	Peru
59.6%	13.8%	7.1%	2	restricted	Philippines
51.5%	27.9%	4.1%	187	banned	Poland
44.2%	19.7%	8.6%	51	restricted	Portugal
–	–	10.1%	7	unknown	Qatar
33.3%	10.8%	6.6%	16	unknown	Romania
58.1%	15.8%	4.2%	13	banned	Russian Federation
–	–	0.9%	–	not regulated	Rwanda
–	–	7.3%	–	unknown	Saint Kitts and Nevis

World Data Table

Country	1 Population Thousands 2002	2 Heart disease		3 Stroke		4 Rheumatic heart disease Number of deaths 2002
		Disability DALYS lost per 1000 population 2002	Mortality Number of deaths 2002	Disability DALYS lost per 1000 population 2003 or latest available data	Mortality Number of deaths 2002	
Saint Lucia	148	6	71	11	120	4
Saint Vincent and Grenadines	119	9	103	10	88	2
Samoa	176	14	117	14	128	3
San Marino	27	5	40	3	26	1
Sao Tome and Principe	157	7	81	10	107	2
Saudi Arabia	23 520	17	16 438	4	3 818	126
Senegal	9 855	10	3 838	12	4 154	355
Serbia and Montenegro	10 535	12	23 610	12	21 756	238
Seychelles	80	7	54	2	15	1
Sierra Leone	4 764	13	2 813	15	3 035	216
Singapore	4 183	7	3 946	3	1 716	39
Slovakia	5 398	12	14 609	5	4 445	131
Slovenia	1 986	6	2 803	6	2 003	87
Solomon Islands	463	12	213	13	220	6
Somalia	9 480	19	6 818	13	4 426	333
South Africa	44 759	9	27 013	11	30 306	792
Spain	40 977	4	45 018	3	34 880	1 738
Sri Lanka	18 910	8	16 297	7	13 348	175
Sudan	32 878	15	28 458	10	16 532	800
Suriname	432	13	397	12	362	4
Swaziland	1 069	8	529	8	499	13
Sweden	8 867	5	20 122	3	9 984	143
Switzerland	7 171	4	10 746	2	4 508	112
Syrian Arab Republic	17 381	13	11 168	11	7 675	1 715
Tajikistan	6 195	23	11 447	7	3 048	419
Tanzania, United Republic of	36 276	10	14 720	12	16 115	439
Thailand	62 193	6	28 425	5	24 810	456
Timor-Leste	739	18	635	10	315	49
Togo	4 801	10	2 474	12	2 675	175
Tonga	103	10	70	12	79	2
Trinidad and Tobago	1 298	15	2 156	10	1 253	23
Tunisia	9 728	15	12 956	6	4 798	298
Turkey	70 318	16	102 552	13	62 782	1 584
Turkmenistan	4 794	34	11 671	7	2 182	221
Tuvalu	10	18	11	20	11	0
Uganda	25 004	10	10 163	11	11 043	288
Ukraine	48 902	28	335 610	13	126 117	3 085
United Arab Emirates	2 937	17	2 235	4	363	16
United Kingdom	59 068	7	120 530	4	59 322	1 712
United States of America	291 038	8	514 450	4	163 768	3 479
Uruguay	3 391	6	3 980	7	3 773	32
Uzbekistan	25 705	24	55 693	12	23 436	1 558
Vanuatu	207	13	120	13	122	3
Venezuela	25 226	10	17 967	5	8 720	208
Viet Nam	80 278	10	66 179	8	58 308	4 210
Yemen	19 315	22	16 217	9	6 464	743
Zambia	10 698	8	4 153	9	4 604	135
Zimbabwe	12 835	8	5 752	10	6 264	158

5 Smoking prevalence Percentage of people 18 years and above who smoke 2003 or latest available data		6 Diabetes Percentage of people aged 20 years and above with diabetes 2000	7 Research Number of publications on cardiovascular disease 1991–2001	8 Policies and legislation Legal status of smoking in government buildings 2004 or latest available data	Country
men	women				
34.6%	5.0%	6.2%	–	restricted	Saint Lucia
34.6%	5.6%	7.3%	–	unknown	Saint Vincent and Grenadines
67.4%	28.8%	6.1%	–	banned	Samoa
–	–	9.2%	–	unknown	San Marino
–	–	0.9%	–	not regulated	Sao Tome and Principe
29.1%	1.2%	9.3%	51	banned	Saudi Arabia
21.2%	1.5%	3.4%	3	not regulated	Senegal
55.5%	51.8%	4.2%	21	not regulated	Serbia & Montenegro
32.5%	15.0%	14.6%	–	unknown	Seychelles
–	–	3.3%	–	unknown	Sierra Leone
23.7%	3.2%	11.4%	76	restricted	Singapore
42.3%	28.0%	3.9%	25	banned	Slovakia
32.7%	20.8%	4.3%	34	restricted	Slovenia
–	–	6.4%	–	restricted	Solomon Islands
–	–	2.7%	–	unknown	Somalia
43.4%	13.9%	3.4%	77	restricted	South Africa
43.9%	31.2%	8.7%	689	restricted	Spain
38.7%	3.1%	5.4%	6	banned	Sri Lanka
27.7%	2.7%	2.9%	–	restricted	Sudan
–	–	3.8%	–	not regulated	Suriname
19.6%	4.9%	2.9%	–	not regulated	Swaziland
21.3%	24.9%	4.3%	654	banned	Sweden
37.6%	28.3%	3.9%	440	restricted	Switzerland
44.0%	16.7%	8.2%	–	banned	Syrian Arab Republic
–	–	3.1%	–	not regulated	Tajikistan
48.9%	7.2%	1.3%	–	not regulated	Tanzania, United Republic of
32.2%	2.7%	3.8%	59	restricted	Thailand
–	–	–	–	unknown	Timor-Leste
–	–	3.1%	2	not regulated	Togo
62.1%	14.2%	6.3%	–	banned	Tonga
–	–	7.3%	5	not regulated	Trinidad and Tobago
52.9%	2.5%	2.9%	8	restricted	Tunisia
51.1%	18.5%	7.3%	578	banned	Turkey
–	–	3.2%	–	banned	Turkmenistan
–	–	6.3%	–	banned	Tuvalu
33.4%	7.1%	1.1%	2	restricted	Uganda
55.5%	14.7%	4.4%	19	restricted	Ukraine
27.6%	4.0%	20.5%	8	restricted	United Arab Emirates
34.6%	34.4%	3.9%	2 667	not regulated	United Kingdom
27.8%	22.3%	8.8%	12 502	restricted	United States of America
39.4%	30.8%	6.8%	2	restricted	Uruguay
28.7%	1.4%	3.2%	1	not regulated	Uzbekistan
47.9%	4.8%	6.9%	–	restricted	Vanuatu
51.9%	20.5%	4.3%	–	unknown	Venezuela
53.2%	3.0%	1.8%	–	banned	Viet Nam
60.0%	29.0%	4.4%	–	unknown	Yemen
21.4%	8.8%	1.6%	–	restricted	Zambia
32.2%	4.6%	2.0%	2	unknown	Zimbabwe

Glossary of terms used in this publication

ACE inhibitors: angiotensin-converting-enzyme inhibitors. Drugs used to treat high blood pressure, and to aid healing after a heart attack.

Angina (angina pectoris): pain or discomfort in the chest that occurs when part of the heart does not receive enough blood. Typically, it is precipitated by effort and relieved by rest.

Angioplasty: a non-invasive surgical procedure used to open up blockages in blood vessels, particularly the coronary arteries that feed the heart. Often performed with either a balloon or a wire mesh (stent).

Anticoagulant: medication that delays the clotting (coagulation) of blood.

Arrhythmia: a change in the regular beat or rhythm of the heart. The heart may seem to skip a beat, or beat irregularly, or beat very fast or very slowly.

Arteriosclerosis: a general term for the hardening of the arteries.

Asymptomatic: without symptoms. This term may apply either to healthy persons or to persons with preclinical (prior to clinical diagnosis) disease in whom symptoms are not yet apparent.

Atherosclerosis: one form of arteriosclerosis, where the hardening and narrowing of the arteries is caused by the slow build-up of fatty deposits on the inside lining.

Atrial fibrillation: a common heart rhythm disorder in which the two small upper chambers of the heart (the atria) quiver instead of beating effectively. This quivering makes the heart less efficient, allows blood to pool and form clots, and predisposes to stroke.

Blood pressure: the force of the blood pushing against the walls of arteries. Blood pressure is given as two numbers: systolic pressure (the pressure while the heart is contracting) and diastolic pressure (the pressure when the heart is resting between contractions).

Body mass index (BMI): a measure of weight in relation to height. It is calculated as weight (in kilograms) divided by the square of height (in metres). A BMI of less than 25 is considered normal, 25–30 is overweight, and greater than 30 defines obesity.

Cardiovascular disease (CVD): any disease of the heart or blood vessels, including stroke and high blood pressure.

Carotid stenosis: narrowing of the carotid arteries, the main arteries in the neck that supply blood to the brain.

Cerebrovascular disease: also called a stroke or the brain equivalent of a heart attack. A condition in which a blood vessel in the brain bursts or is clogged by a blood clot, leading to inadequate blood supply to the brain and death of brain cells.

Cholesterol: a waxy substance that circulates in the bloodstream.

Cholesterol plaques: deposits of fat, cholesterol, cellular waste products, calcium and other substances that build up on the inner lining of an artery.

Congestive heart failure: a condition in which the heart cannot pump enough blood to meet the needs of the body's other organs.

Coronary artery bypass surgery (CABG): A type of heart surgery that re-routes blood around clogged arteries – or "bypasses" them – to improve the supply of blood and oxygen to the heart.

Coronary heart disease: heart disease in which the coronary arteries are narrowed and the supply of blood and oxygen to the heart therefore decreased. Also called coronary artery disease or ischaemic heart disease. It includes heart attack and angina.

Developing country, high mortality: a developing country with high child mortality and high or very high adult mortality.

Developing country, low mortality: a developing country with low child mortality and low adult mortality.

Diabetes mellitus: a chronic disease due to either insulin deficiency or resistance to insulin action or both, and associated with hyperglycaemia (elevated blood glucose levels).

Direct costs: costs associated with an illness that can be attributed to a medical service, procedure, medication, etc., such as X-ray examination, pharmaceutical drugs (for example, insulin), surgery, or a clinic visit.

Disability adjusted life years (DALYs): a measure of overall burden of a disease by combining the years of potential life lost due to premature death and the years of productive life lost due to the disability. One DALY is one lost year of healthy life.

Epidemic: the occurrence in a community or region of cases of an illness, specific health-related behaviour, or other health-related events clearly in excess of what would normally be expected.

Health: a state of complete physical, mental, and social well-being and not merely the absence of disease or infirmity.

HDL (high-density lipoprotein) cholesterol: the so-called "good cholesterol". HDL helps remove cholesterol from the blood vessels. High levels of blood HDL protect against heart disease.

Heart attack (myocardial infarction): death of part of the heart muscle as a result of a coronary artery becoming completely blocked, usually by a blood clot (thrombus), resulting in lack of blood flow to the heart muscle and therefore loss of needed oxygen.

Heart failure: see Congestive heart failure.

High blood pressure: a systolic blood pressure of 140 mmHg or greater or a diastolic pressure of 90 mmHg or greater.

Homocysteine: an amino acid produced by the body. Elevated levels of homocysteine in the blood can damage blood vessels and disrupt normal blood clotting, and possibly increase the risk of heart attack, stroke, and peripheral vascular disease.

Indirect costs: costs associated with an illness that occur because an individual or family members cannot work at their usual jobs, because of premature death, sickness, or disability.

Ischaemic heart disease: see Coronary heart disease.

LDL (low-density lipoprotein) cholesterol: the so-called "bad cholesterol". High levels of LDL put people at risk of heart attack.

Lipid: fat or fat-like substance, such as cholesterol, present in blood and body tissues.

MET: metabolic equivalent; a measure of energy expenditure. One MET/min is the amount of energy expended while sitting quietly at rest for one minute.

Obesity: a condition characterized by excessive body fat. Usually defined as a body mass index greater than 30.

Peripheral vascular disease: disease of certain blood vessels outside the heart or disease of the lymph vessels, for example the arteries supplying the limbs, which leads to inadequate blood supply and claudication (intermittent pain on exercise such as walking).

Physical activity: bodily movement that substantially increases energy expenditure.

Premature death: death that occurs at an age earlier than the average life expectancy for the population.

Primary prevention: a strategy that helps to prevent the onset of a disease or condition in people who are at risk but do not already have the disease or condition. Examples are promotion of exercise in the general population, smoking prevention in young people, and also the treatment and control of high blood pressure as a strategy for primary prevention of stroke.

Rheumatic heart disease: damage to the heart valves and other heart structures from inflammation and scarring caused by rheumatic fever. Rheumatic fever begins with a sore throat due to streptococcal infection.

Secondary prevention: a strategy that helps to prevent recurrent disease or complications in people who already have the disease. For example, the use of a daily dose of aspirin by heart attack survivors is an effective strategy for preventing a second heart attack.

Sedentary: denotes a person who is relatively inactive and has a lifestyle characterized by a lot of sitting.

Stent: a device used to support tissues while healing takes place. A stent can keep "tube-shaped" structures, such as blood vessels, open after a surgical procedure. An intraluminal coronary artery stent is a small, self-expanding, stainless steel mesh tube, which is placed within a coronary artery to keep the vessel open.

Stroke: the brain equivalent of a heart attack. A condition in which a blood vessel in the brain bursts (haemorrhagic stroke) or is clogged (embolic or ischaemic stroke) by a blood clot. This leads to inadequate blood supply to the brain and death of the brain cells, and usually results in temporary or permanent neurological deficits.

Transient ischaemic attack (TIA): small stroke-like event, which resolves in a day or less. It is often a warning sign of an impending stroke.

Triglyceride: the chemical form in which most fat exists in food and in the body.

Sources

PART 1 CARDIOVASCULAR DISEASE

1 Types of cardiovascular disease

Deaths from cardiovascular diseases
Mortality and burden of disease estimates for
countries provided by Colin Mathers (Evidence and
Information for Policy, WHO) from analyses
prepared for *The World Health Report 2003*.

Global deaths from CVD
World Health Organization. *The World Health Report
2003: shaping the future*. Geneva, WHO, 2003,
Annex Table 2:156.

Clipboard
WHO. *The World Health Report 2003: shaping the
future*. Geneva, WHO, 2003, Annex Table 2:156.

2 Rheumatic fever and rheumatic heart disease

Map: Deaths from rheumatic heart disease
Mortality and burden of disease estimates for
countries provided by Colin Mathers (Evidence and
Information for Policy, WHO) from analyses
prepared for *The World Health Report 2003*.

Rheumatic heart disease in children
Carapetis JR. The current evidence for the burden of
group A streptococcal diseases. *A review of WHO
activities in, the burden of, and the evidence for strategies
to control group A streptococcal diseases*. Geneva,
WHO, 2004.

**Deaths from rheumatic fever and rheumatic
heart disease in the Aboriginal and non-
Aboriginal populations of Australia**
Carapetis JR, Currie BJ. Mortality due to acute
rheumatic fever and rheumatic heart disease in the
Northern Territory: a preventable cause of death in
Aboriginal people. *Australian and New Zealand journal
of public health*, 1999, 23:159–163.

Clipboard
*Rheumatic fever and rheumatic heart disease: report of a
WHO Expert Committee*. Geneva, WHO, 2003 (WHO
Technical Report Series, No. 923).

Text
Stollerman GH. Rheumatic fever in the 21st century.
Clinics in infectious diseases, 2001, 33:806–814.

Treating acute rheumatic fever. *British medical journal*,
2003, 327:631–63 (editorial).

WHO. *The World Health Report 2003: shaping the
future*. Geneva, WHO, 2003, Annex Table 2:156.

Veasy LG, Hill HR. Immunologic and clinical
correlations in rheumatic fever and rheumatic heart
disease. *Pediatric infectious diseases journal*, 1997,
16:400–407.

PART 2 RISK FACTORS

3 Risk factors

Leading risk factors
WHO. Leading 10 selected risk factors as percentage
cause of disease burden measured in DALYs. *The
World Health Report 2002: reducing risks, promoting
healthy life*. Geneva, WHO, 2002, 162.

Contributory factors
WHO. Quantifying selected major risks to health.
*The World Health Report 2002: reducing risks, promoting
healthy life*. Geneva, WHO, 2002, 57–61.

Clipboard
Beaglehole R, Magnus P. The search for new risk
factors for coronary heart disease: occupational therapy
for epidemiologists? *International journal of epidemiology*,
2002, 31(6):1117–22; author reply 1134–5.

Text
Inter-Society Commission for Heart Disease
Resources A: Primary prevention of the
atherosclerotic diseases. *Circulation*, 1970,
42:A55–A95.

4 Risk factors start in childhood and youth

Maps: Early starters; Clipboard
Global Youth Collaborating Group. Special report: Differences in worldwide tobacco use by gender: findings from the Global Youth Tobacco Survey. *Journal of school health*, 2003, 73(6):207–215. Detailed country information available at: http://www.cdc.gov/tobacco/global/GYTS.htm

Overweight trends in the USA
CDC, National Center for Health Statistics. Health, United States, 2003 with Chartbook on trends in the health of Americans. Hyattsville, MD, 2003. BMI at or above the sex-age-specific 95th percentile http://www.cdc.gov/nchs/data/hus/tables/2003/03hus069.pdf

Overweight youth
Lissau I, Overpeck MD, Ruan WJ, Due P, Holstein BE, Hedinger M, and the Health Behaviour in School-aged Children Working Group. Body mass index and overweight in adolescents in 13 European countries, Israel, and the United States. *Archives of pediatric and adolescent medicine*, 2004, 158:27–33. Table 3. Prevalence of BMI at or above the 95th percentile (overweight) by sex (self-reported).

Wow: USA
Kimm SYS et al. Decline in physical activity in black girls and white girls during adolescence. *New England journal of medicine*, 2002, 347:709–15.

Clipboard
Overweight: WHO Fact Sheet, Global Strategy on Diet, Physical Activity and Health. Obesity and overweight. Geneva, WHO, 2003 http://www.who.int/hpr/gs.facts.shtml

Text
Zimmet P. The burden of type 2 diabetes: are we doing enough? *Diabetes and metabolism*, 2003, 29(4 Pt 2):6S9–6S18.

Kitagawa T, Owada M, Urakami T, Yamauchi K. Increased incidence of non-insulin dependent diabetes mellitus among Japanese schoolchildren correlates with an increased intake of animal protein and fat. *Clinical pediatrics (Philadelphia)*, 1998, 37(2):111–115.

Likitmaskul S, Kiattisathavee P, Chaichanwatanakul K, Punnakanta L, Angsusingha K, Tuchinda C. Increasing prevalence of type 2 diabetes mellitus in Thai children and adolescents associated with increasing prevalence of obesity. *Journal of pediatric endocrinology and metabolism*, 2003, 16(1):71–77.

Berenson GS, Srinivasan SR, Bao W, Newman WP 3rd, Tracy RE, Wattigney WA. Association between multiple cardiovascular risk factors and atherosclerosis in children and young adults. The Bogalusa Heart Study. *New England journal of medicine*, 1998, 338(23):1650–1656.

5 Risk factor: blood pressure

Maps: Blood Pressure
WHO Global NCD InfoBase [online database]. Geneva, WHO, 2004 http://www.who.int/ncd_surveillance/infobase/

High blood pressure in the USA
Trends, USA, 1960–2000; Health, United States 2002; Table 68. Hypertension among persons 20 years of age and over, according to sex, age, race, and Hispanic origin: United States, 1960–62,1971–74, 1976–80, 1988–94, and 1999–2000. Referencing Centers for Disease Control and Prevention, National Center for Health Statistics, National Health and Nutrition Examination Survey, Hispanic Health and Nutrition Examination Survey (1982–84), and National Health Examination Survey (1960–62) http://www.cdc.gov/nchs/data/hus/hus02.pdf

Blood pressure changes with age in the Gambia
van der Sande MA, Bailey R, Faal H et al. Nationwide prevalence study of hypertension and related non-communicable diseases in The Gambia. *Tropical medicine and international health*, 1997, 2(11):1039–1048.

Blood pressure in India
Singh RB, Suh IL, Singh V. et al. Hypertension and stroke in Asia: prevalence, control and strategies in developing countries for prevention. *Journal of human hypertension*, 2000, 14:749–763.

High blood pressure by years of education in South Africa
South Africa Demographic and Health Survey 1998
http://www.doh.gov.za/facts/1998/sadhs98/

Text
Vasan RS, Larson MG, Leip EP, Evans JC, O'Donnell CJ, Kannel WB, Levy D. Impact of high-normal blood pressure on the risk of cardiovascular disease. *New England journal of medicine*, 2001, 345:1291–1297.

World Hypertension League. The high blood pressure/heart failure link: a new concern for older Americans
http://www.mco.edu/org/whl/hrtfail.html

Huxley R, Neil A, Collins R. Unravelling the fetal origins hypothesis: is there really an inverse association between birthweight and subsequent blood pressure? *Lancet*, 2002, 360:659–665.

Systolic blood pressure. *British medical journal*, 2002, 325:917–918 (editorial).

Sleight P. Fact sheet: isolated hypertension (ISH). World Hypertension League
http://www.mco.edu/org/whl/isyshype.html

Weinberger MH, Miller JZ, Luft FC, Grim CE, Fineberg NS. Definitions and characteristics of sodium sensitivity and blood pressure resistance. *Hypertension*, 1986, 8(2):127–134.

He J, Ogden LG, Vupputuri S, Bazzano LA, Loria C, Whelton PK. Dietary sodium intake and subsequent risk of cardiovascular disease in overweight adults. *Journal of the American Medical Association*, 1999, 282:2027–2034.

6 Risk factor: lipids

Map: Cholesterol
WHO Global NCD InfoBase [online database]. Geneva, WHO
http://www.who.int/ncd_surveillance/infobase/

Current recommended lipid levels
De Backer G, Ambrosioni E, Borch-Johnsen K et al.; Third Joint Force of European and other Societies on Cardiovascular Disease and Prevention in Clinical Practice. European guidelines on cardiovascular disease prevention in clinical practice. *Atherosclerosis*, 2003, 171(1):145–155.

Third Report of the National Cholesterol Education Program (NCEP) Expert Panel on Detection, Evaluation, and Treatment of High Blood Cholesterol in Adults (Adult Treatment Panel III) final report. *Circulation*, 2002, 106:3143–3421
http://circ.ahajournals.org/cgi/reprint/106/25/3143.pdf

Trends in cholesterol levels in Beijing, China
Tolonen H, Kuulasmaa K, Ruokokoski. MONICA population survey data book. 2000 (data from 1984–1993). Zhao Dong, personal communication (data from 1996–1999).

Wow: USA
American Heart Foundation. About cholesterol
http://www.americanheart.org/presenter.jhtml?identifier=185

Clipboard
WHO. *The World Health Report 2002: reducing risks, promoting healthy life*. Geneva, WHO, 2002.

Text
American Heart Foundation. About cholesterol
http://www.americanheart.org/

7 Risk factor: tobacco

Maps: Smoking prevalence
WHO Global NCD InfoBase [online database]. Geneva, WHO
http://www.who.int/ncd_surveillance/infobase/

Cardiovascular risks of smoking
Price JF, Mowbray PI, Lee AJ, Rumley A, Lowe GD, Fowkes FG. Smoking and cardiovascular risk factors in the development of cardiovascular disease and coronary artery disease: Edinburgh Artery Study. *European heart journal*, 1999, 20:344–353.

Prescott E, Hippe M, Schnohr P, Hein HO, Vestbo J. Smoking and risk of myocardial infarction in women and men: longitudinal population study. *British medical journal*, 1998, 316:1043–1047.

Smoking and stroke: a causative role. Heavy smokers with hypertension benefit most from stopping. *British medical journal*, 1998, 317:962–963 (editorial).

Cole CW, Hill GB, Farzad E, Bouchard A, Moher D, Rody K, Shea B. Cigarette smoking and peripheral arterial occlusive disease. *Surgery*, 1993, 114(4):753–756; discussion, 756–757.

Lederle FA, Johnson GR, Wilson SE et al. Prevalence and associations of abdominal aortic aneurysm detected through screening. Aneurysm Detection and Management (ADAM) Veterans Affairs Cooperative Study Group. *Annals of internal medicine*, 1997, 126(6):441–449.

Smoking and urology: male fertility and sexuality dysfunctions. *Cigarettes: what the warning label doesn't tell you: the first comprehensive guide to the health consequences of smoking*. New York. The American Council on Science and Health, 1996, Chapter 11:95–100.

Smoking harms men. *Sydney Morning Herald*, 24 March 1997, 3 (quoting *Australian and New Zealand journal of medicine*).

Cardiovascular risks of passive smoking

Panagiotakos DB, Pitsavos C, Chrysohoou C, Skoumas J, Masoura C, Toutouzas P, Stefanadis C. Effect of exposure to secondhand smoke on markers of inflammation: the ATTICA study. *American journal of medicine*, 2004, 116(3):145–150.

Bonita R, Duncan J, Truelsen T, Jackson RT, Beaglehole R. Passive smoking as well as active smoking increases the risk of stroke. *Tobacco control*, 1999, 8:156–161.

International Consultation on Environmental Tobacco Smoke (ETS) and Child Health, 11–14 January 1999. Geneva, WHO, 1999 (WHO/NCD/TFI//99.10).

Smokers don't know the risks of heart attack

Ayanian JZ, Cleary PD. Perceived risks of heart disease and cancer among cigarette smokers. *Journal of the American Medical Association*, 1999, 281:1019–1021.

Wow: USA

National Cancer Institute. *Health effects of exposure to environmental tobacco smoke: the report of the California Environmental Protection Agency*. Bethesda, MD, US Department of Health and Human Services, National Institutes of Health, National Cancer Institute, 1999 (Smoking and Tobacco Control Monograph no. 10; NIH Pub. No. 99–4645).

Wow: China

Smoking and health in China. *1996 National Prevalence Survey of Smoking Pattern*. Beijing, China Science and Technology Press, undated, 89.

Text

English JP, Willius FA, Berkson J. Tobacco and coronary disease. *Journal of the American Medical Association*, 1940, 115:1327–1329.

Smoking study reveals grim disease risks. Australian Associated Press, 20 May 2002 http://news.ninemsn.com.au/Health/story_31927. asp?MSID=6d40353f6b864cd7806381801f7fdc0a

Bonita R, Duncan J, Truelsen T, Jackson RT, Beaglehole R. Passive smoking as well as active smoking increases the risk of acute stroke. *Tobacco control*, 1999, 8:156–160.

Lehr HA, Weyrich AS, Saetzle RK et al. Vitamin C blocks inflammatory platelet-activating factor mimetics created by cigarette smoking. *Journal of clinical investigation*, 1997, 99(10):2358–2364.

Davis JW, Shelton L, Watanabe IS, Arnold J. Passive smoking affects endothelium and platelets. *Archives of internal medicine*, 1989, 149(2):386–389.

McBride PE. The health consequences of smoking: cardivascular disease. *Medical clinics of North America*, 1992, 76:333–353.

Aronow W. Effect of passive smoking on angina pectoris. *New England journal of medicine*, 1978, 299:21–24.

Humphries SE, Talmud PJ, Hawe E, Bolla M, Day INM, Miller GJ. Apolipoprotein E4 and coronary heart disease in middle-aged men who smoke: a prospective study. *Lancet*, 2001, 358:115–119. *Gene linked to heart disease risk*. BBC online, 13 July 2001 http://www.bbc.co.uk

Prescott E, Scharling H, Osler M, Schnohr P. Importance of light smoking and inhalation habits on risk of myocardial infarction and all cause mortality. A 22 year follow up of 12 149 men and women in The Copenhagen City Heart Study. *Journal of epidemiology and community health*, 2002, 56:702–706 http://jech.bmjjournals.com/cgi/content/abstract/56/9/702

Willett WC, Green A, Stampfer MJ et al. Relative and absolute excess risks of coronary heart disease among women who smoke cigarettes. *New England journal of medicine*, 1987, 317:1303–1309.

8 Risk factor: physical inactivity

Map: Physical activity levels
Non-EU countries

Unpublished preliminary analysis of the World Health Survey 2002–2003. Geneva, WHO.

Rütten A et al. Using different physical activity measurements in eight European countries. Results of the European Physical Activity Surveillance System (EUPASS) time series survey. *Public health nutrition*, 2003, 6(4):371–376.

World Health Survey. Eurobarometer: International Physical Activity Questionnaire (IPAQ). Geneva, WHO http://www.who.int/ncd_surveillance/infobase/

EU countries

Rütten A, Abu-Omar K. Prevalence of physical activity in the European Union. *Sozial- und Präventivmedizin/Social and Preventative Medicine*, 2004, 49(4).

World Health Survey. Eurobarometer: International Physical Activity Questionnaire (IPAQ). Geneva, WHO http://www.who.int/ncd_surveillance/infobase/

Sitting

Rütten A et al. Using different physical activity measurements in eight European countries. Results of the European Physical Activity Surveillance System (EUPASS) time series survey. *Public health nutrition*, 2003, 6(4):371–376.

Physical activity

Department of Health, Hong Kong. *Fact sheet on physical activity* http://www.info.gov.hk/dh/do_you_k/eng/exercise.htm

Physical inactivity by social class in India

Singh RB, Sharma JP, Rastogi V, Niaz MA, Singh NK. Prevalence and determinants of hypertension in the Indian social class and heart survey. *Journal of human hypertension*, 1997, 11:51–56.

Singapore keeps moving

National Health Survey 1998. Singapore, Epidemiology and Disease Control Department, Ministry of Health, 1998.

Transport

American Automobile Manufacturers Association (AAMA). Motor vehicle facts and figures 1996. *Proceed with caution: growth in the global motor vehicle fleet*. Washington DC, World Resources Institute, 1996, 44–47 http://www.wri.org/trends/autos2.html

The global fleet

American Automobile Manufacturers Association (AAMA). World motor vehicle data 1993; and Motor vehicle facts and figures 1996. *Proceed with caution: growth in the global motor vehicle fleet*. Washington, DC, World Resources Institute, 1996 http://www.wri.org/trends/autos2.html

Wow: Being physically active…; Text

Bull FC, Armstrong T, Dixon T, Ham S, Neiman A, Pratt M. Physical inactivity. Ezzati M, Lopez A, Rodgers A, Murray C, eds. *Comparative quantification of health risks: global and regional burden of disease due to selected major risk factors*. Geneva, WHO, 2004 (in press).

Wow: Worldwide, physical inactivity…
The World Health Report 2002: reducing risks, promoting healthy life. Geneva, WHO, 2002:61.

Wow: In 1997, in China…
Matters of scale: November/ December 1997. Driving up CO_2 http://www.worldwatch.org/pubs/mag/1997/106/mos/

Wow: 25% of the world's cars…
Renner M. Live online discussions. Five hundred million cars, one planet – Who's going to give? 8 August 2003 http://www.worldwatch.org/live/discussion/83/

Text
World Heart Federation. A global embrace for World Heart Day. Message from the President, 29 Sept 2002 http://www.worldheartday.org/WHDArchive/whd2002/news/news.asp#

Kujala UM, Kaprio J, Sarna S, Koskenvuo M. Relationship of leisure-time physical activity and mortality: the Finnish twin cohort. Journal of the American Medical Association, 1998, 279:440–444.

HeartBytes. Reduce heart disease risk: encourage and prescribe exercise for your patients. http://www.medscape.com/viewarticle/470115?mpid=25341

Cervero R. Shapeless, spread out, skipped over and scattershot – sprawl sweeps the globe. The World Paper, http://www.worldpaper.com/2000/mar2000/cervero.html

9 Risk factor: obesity

Maps: Body mass index
WHO Global NCD InfoBase [online database]. Geneva, WHO http://www.who.int/ncd_surveillance/infobase/

Food consumption
Diet, nutrition and the prevention of chronic diseases: report of a Joint WHO/FAO Expert Consultation. Geneva, WHO, 2003 (WHO Technical Report Series No. 916): Table 1:15. Data from: Popkin BM. The shift in stages of the nutritional transition in the developing world differs from past experiences! Public health nutrition, 2002, 5:205–214.

Apple shape at higher risk of CVD than pear shape
Lakka HM, Lakka TA, Tuomilehto J, Salonen JT. Abdominal obesity is associated with increased risk of acute coronary events in men. European heart journal, 2002,23:706–713 (cited in Sowers JR. Obesity as a cardiovascular risk factor. American journal of medicine, 2003, 115(8A):37S–41S).

Isomaa B, Almgren P, Tuomi T, et al. Cardiovascular morbidity and mortality associated with the metabolic syndrome. Diabetes care, 2001, 24:683–689 (cited in Sowers JR. Obesity as a cardiovascular risk factor. American journal of medicine, 2003, 115(8A):37S–41S).

Overweight and obesity: defining overweight and obesity http://www.cdc.gov/nccdphp/dnpa/obesity/defining.htm

Wow: Thailand
Associated Press in Bangkok. Thailand: Chubby nights soothe the heavyweight clubbers. South China Morning Post, 12 September 2002, 11.

Text
WHO expert consultation. Appropriate body-mass index for Asian populations and its implications for policy and intervention strategies. Lancet, 2004, 363:157–63.

Eckel RH, Krauss RM. American Heart Association call to action: obesity as a major risk factor for coronary heart disease. Circulation, 1998, 97:2099–2100.

WHO. The World Health Report 2002: reducing risks, promoting healthy life. Geneva, WHO, 2002.

Peeters A, Barendregt JJ, Willekens F, Mackenbach JP, Mamun AA, Bonneux L. Obesity in adulthood and its consequences for life expectancy: a life table analysis. Annals of internal medicine, 2003, 138:24–32.

The catastrophic failures of public health. Lancet, 2004, 363(9411):157–63 (editorial)).

Buncombe A. American undertakers offer 'super-size' coffins as population piles on the pounds. *The Independent*, 29 September 2003 http://news.independent.co.uk/world/americas/story.jsp?story=448034

Fast food takeaways China. BBC online, 1999 http://news.bbc.co.uk/hi/english/health/newsid_364000/364273.stm

Easen N. *Asia falls foul to fat.* CNN, 21 Feb 2002 http://www.cnn.com/2002/WORLD/asiapcf/auspac/02/21/asia.obesity/?related

Associated Press. New Zealand. *Boarding pass and scales, please – NZ weighs the trend for heavier passenger loads. South China Morning Post*, 4 October 2003, A10.

10 Risk factor: diabetes

Map: Prevalence of diabetes; Diabetes prevalence and trends; Clipboard

Wild S, Roglic G, Green A, Sicree R, King H. Global prevalence of diabetes. Estimates for the year 2000 and projections for 2030. *Diabetes care*, 2004, 27:1047–1053.

Text

International Diabetes Federation http://www.idf.org/home/index.cfm?node=264

11 Risk factor: socioeconomic status

Prevalence of CVD risk factors by education in Canada

Choiniere R, Lafontaine P, Edwards AC. Distribution of cardiovascular disease risk factors by socioeconomic status among Canadian adults. *Canadian Medical Association journal*, 2000, 162(9 Suppl):S13–24. Note: Definitions used: Physical inactivity: leisure exercise less than once per week during previous month. Elevated cholesterol: ≥5.2 mmol/l after fasting 8 hours or more.

The CVD mortality gap in the USA

Singh GK, Siahpush M. Increasing inequalities in all-cause and cardiovascular mortality among US adults aged 25–64 years by area and socioeconomic status, 1969–1998. *International journal of epidemiology*, 2002, 31(3):600–613.

Prevalence of high blood pressure by income in Trinidad and Tobago

Gulliford MC, Mahabir D, Rocke B. Socioeconomic inequality in blood pressure and its determinants: cross-sectional data from Trinidad and Tobago. *Journal of human hypertension*, 2004, 18:61–70.

Education level and obesity in Italy

Giampaoli S, Palmieri L, Dima F, Pilotto L, Vescio MF, Vanuzzo D. Socioeconomic aspects and cardiovascular risk factors: experience at the Cardiovascular Epidemiologic Observatory. *Italian heart journal*, 2001, 2(3 Suppl):294–302.

Smoking and occupation in Uganda

Uganda Demographic and Health Survey 2000–2001.

Smoking by years of education in South Africa

South Africa Demographic and Health Survey (SADHS) 1998.

Income and obesity in Saudi Arabia

Al-Nuaim AA et al. Overweight and obesity in Saudi Arabian adult population, role of socio-demographic variables. *Journal of community health*, 1997, 22(3):211–23.

Prevalence of diabetes by income in India

Ramachandran A, Snehalatha C, Kapur A et al. Diabetes Epidemiology Study Group in India (DESI). High prevalence of diabetes and impaired glucose tolerance in India: National Urban Diabetes Survey. *Diabetologia*, 2001, 44(9):1094–101.

Wow: Canada

Evenson B. When rich and poor kids eat the same diet, poor ones get fatter. *ProCOR*, 12 September 2003.

Clipboard

Steptoe A, Feldman PJ, Kunz S, Owen N, Willemsen G, Marmot M. Stress responsivity and socioeconomic status: a mechanism for increased cardiovascular disease risk? *European heart journal*, 2002, 23(22):1757–63.

Text

Terris M. The development and prevention of cardiovascular disease risk factors: socioenvironmental influences. *Preventive medicine*, 1999, 29(6 Pt 2):S11–17.

Pickering T. Cardiovascular pathways: socioeconomic status and stress effects on hypertension and cardiovascular function. *Annals of the New York Academy of Sciences*, 1999, 896:262–277.

Rao SV, Kaul P, Newby K et al. Poverty, process of care, and outcome in acute coronary syndrome. *Journal of the American College of Cardiology*, 2003, 41:1948–54.

12 Women: a special case?

Smoking
Prescott E, Hippe M, Schnohr P, Hein HO, Vestbo J. Smoking and risk of myocardial infarction in women and men: longitudinal population study. *British medical journal*, 1998, 316:1043–1047.

No time to walk
Clark J. News roundup: Women too busy to exercise. *British medical journal*, 2003, 326:467.

Walking reduces coronary heart disease
Lee IM, Rexrode KM, Cook NR, Manson JE, Buring JE. Physical activity and coronary heart disease in women. Is "no pain, no gain" passé? *Journal of the American Medical Association*, 2001, 285:1447–1454.

Hormone replacement therapy
Trevisan MM. Hormone replacement therapy. *Global Symposium on Cardiovascular Prevention, Marbella, Spain*, 11–13 April 2003.

Clipboard
WHO. *The World Health Report 2003: Shaping the future*. Geneva, WHO, 2003: Annex Table 2.

Text
Kmietowicz Z. News roundup: Women fail to recognise risk of heart disease. *British medical journal*, 2003, 326:355.

Ulmer H, Kelleher C, Diem G, Concin H. Why Eve is not Adam: prospective follow-up in 149650 women and men of cholesterol and other risk factors related to cardiovascular and all-cause mortality. *Journal of women's health (Larchmount)*, 2004, 13(1):41–53.

Lerner DJ, Kannel WB. Patterns of coronary heart disease morbidity and mortality in the sexes: a 26-year follow-up of the Framingham population. *American heart journal*, 1986, 111:383–390.

McKinlay JB. Some contributions from the social system to gender inequalities in heart disease. *Journal of health and social behaviour*, 1996, 37:1–26.

Giles WH, Anda RF, Casper ML, Escobedo LG, Taylor HA. Race and sex differences in rates of invasive cardiac procedures in US hospitals: data from the National Hospital Discharge Survey. *Archives of internal medicine*, 1995, 155:318–324.

Dustan HP. Coronary artery disease in women. *Canadian journal of cardiology*, 1990, 6(Suppl B):19B–21B.

Lehmann JB, Wehner PS, Lehmann CU, Savory LM. Gender bias in the evaluation of chest pain in the emergency department. *American journal of cardiology*, 1996, 77:641–644.

Roquer J, Campello AR, Gomis M. Sex differences in first-ever acute stroke. *Stroke*, 2003, 34(7):1581–1585.

Adams KF Jr, Sueta CA, Gheorghiade M, O'Connor CM, Schwartz TA, Koch GG, Uretsky B, Swedberg K, McKenna W, Soler-Soler J, Califf RM. Gender differences in survival in advanced heart failure. Insights from the FIRST study. *Circulation*, 1999, 99(14):1816–1821.

Mosca L et al. Evidence-based guidelines for cardiovascular disease prevention in women. *Circulation*, 2004, 109:672–693.

PART 3 THE BURDEN

13 Global burden of coronary heart disease

Map: Healthy years of life lost to coronary heart disease
Mortality and burden of disease estimates for countries provided by Colin Mathers (Evidence and Information for Policy, WHO) from analyses prepared for *The World Health Report 2003*.

Disease burden in men; in women
WHO. *The World Health Report 2003: Shaping the future*. Geneva, WHO, 2003.

Clipboard; Text
Ounpuu S, Anand S, Yusuf S. The global burden of cardiovascular disease. Medscape cardiology, 24 January 2002
http://www.medscape.com/viewarticle/420877?WebLogicSession=Pj4P2wsr611rYWKbLSDskpUMbsjmJxtWvxSNaGHCVd2ranocYJpC|42976445789882471 33/184161393/6/7001/7001/7002/7002/7001/-1

Text
Nayha S. Cold and the risk of cardiovascular diseases. *A review. International journal of circumpolar health*, 2002, 61(4):373–380.

14 Deaths from coronary heart disease

Map: Deaths from coronary heart disease
Mortality and burden of disease estimates for countries provided by Colin Mathers (Evidence and Information for Policy, WHO) from analyses prepared for *The World Health Report 2003*.

Deaths from coronary heart disease compared with other causes
WHO. *The World Health Report 2003: Shaping the future*. Geneva, WHO, 2003, Table 1.3:17.

Change of heart
British Heart Foundation Statistics database.
1. Mortality. Table 1.5
http://www.heartstats.org

Wow: 3.8 million men…
WHO. *The World Health Report 2003: Shaping the future*. Geneva, WHO, 2003, Annex Table 2:154–159.

Text
Ounpuu S, Anand S, Yusuf S. The global burden of cardiovascular disease. *Medscape cardiology*, 24 January 2002
http://www.medscape.com/viewarticle/420877?WebLogicSession=Pj4P2wsr611rYWKbLSDskpUMbsjmJxtWvxSNaGHCVd2ranocYJpC|42976445789882471 33/184161393/6/7001/7001/7002/7002/7001/-1

Khot UN, Khot MB, Bajzer CT et al. Prevalence of conventional risk factors in patients with coronary heart disease. *Journal of the American Medical Association*, 2003, 290:898–904.

Chambless L, Keil U, Dobson A, Mahonen M, Kuulasmaa K, Rajakangas AM, Lowel H, Tunstall-Pedoe H. Population versus clinical view of case fatality from acute coronary heart disease: results from the WHO MONICA Project 1985–1990. Multinational MONItoring of Trends and Determinants in CArdiovascular Disease. *Circulation*, 1997, 96(11):3849–59.

15 Global burden of stroke

Map: Healthy years of life lost to stroke
Mortality and burden of disease estimates for countries provided by Colin Mathers (Evidence and Information for Policy, WHO) from analyses prepared for *The World Health Report 2003*.

Stroke in young people
Jacobs BS, Boden-Albala B, Lin IF, Sacco RL. Stroke in the young in the northern Manhattan stroke study. *Stroke*, 2002, 33(12):2789–93.

Oral contraceptives
Lidegaard Ø, Kreiner S. Contraceptives and cerebral thrombosis: a five-year national case-control study. *Contraception*, 2002, 65:197–205.

Wow: United Kingdom
Wise J. News: New clinical guidelines for stroke published. *British medical journal*, 2000, 320:823.

Wow: Stroke burden, 2020
Murray CJL, Lopez AD. *The global burden of disease*. Boston, Harvard School of Public Health (for WHO and the World Bank), 1996, Table 17i:830.

Clipboard
Chobanian AV, Bakris GL, Black HR et al. The Seventh Report of the Joint National Committee on Prevention, Detection, Evaluation, and Treatment of High Blood Pressure: The JNC 7 Report. *Journal of the American Medical Association*, 2003, 289:2560–2572.

Text
McCarron P, Davey Smith G, Okasha M, McEwen J. Blood pressure in young adulthood and mortality from cardiovascular disease. *Lancet*, 2000, 355:1430–31.

Adams RJ, McKie VC, Brambilla D et al. Stroke prevention trial in sickle cell anemia. Control clinical trials, *New England journal of medicine*, 1998, 19:110–129.

Bonita R, Scragg R, Stewart A, Jackson R, Beaglehole R. Cigarette smoking and risk of premature stroke in men and women. *British medical journal*, 1986, 293:6–8.

Lip GYH, Kamath S, Hart RG. Clinical review: ABC of antithrombotic therapy. Antithrombotic therapy for cerebrovascular disorders. *British medical journal*, 2002, 325:1161–1163.

16 Deaths from stroke

Map: Struck down
Mortality and burden of disease estimates for countries provided by Colin Mathers (Evidence and Information for Policy, WHO) from analyses prepared for *The World Health Report 2003*.

Predictors of death from stroke in Italy
Mazza A, Pessina AC, Pavei A, Scarpa R, Tikhonoff V, Casiglia E. Predictors of stroke mortality in elderly people from the general population. The CArdiovascular STudy in the ELderly. *European journal of epidemiology*, 2001, 17(12):1097–1104.

Stroke compared with other causes of death; Wow: Worldwide…
WHO. *The World Health Report 2003: Shaping the future*. Geneva, WHO, 2003, Annex Table 2:154–159.

Wow: USA
American Stroke Association
http://www.strokeassociation.org/presenter.jhtml?identifier=1033

Clipboard
Lip GYH, Kamath S, Hart RG. Clinical review: ABC of antithrombotic therapy. Antithrombotic therapy for cerebrovascular disorders. *British medical journal*, 2002, 325:1161–1163.

Text
The Stroke Association, United Kingdom. *Stroke prevention programmes*
http://www.stroke.org.uk/Campaign/prevention.htm

Mensah GA. Global burden of hypertension: good news and bad news. *Cardiology clinics*, 2002, 20:181–186.

Heller RF, Langhorne P, James E. Improving stroke outcomes: the benefits of increasing availability of technology. *Bulletin of the WHO*, 2000, 78:1337–1343.

17 Economic costs

Global costs of smoking
WHO. World No Tobacco Day 2004
http://www.who.int/tobacco/areas/communications/events/wntd/2004/en/

Global costs of heart disease medication
Kmietowicz Z. News: WHO warns of heart disease threat to developing world. *British medical journal*, 2002, 325:853.

Global costs of diabetes
International Diabetes Federation
http://www.idf.org/home/index.cfm?unode=3B9691D3-C026-2FD3-87B7FA0B63432BA3

Latin America and the Caribbean
PAHO cites impact of diabetes in Latin America
http://www.unwire.org

USA, Australia, Europe
Reuters. Asia-Pacific Type 2 Diabetes Policy Group: spread of diabetes in Asia alarms experts. *South China Morning Post*, 1 May 2002, 10.

USA
Runners beat around the Bush. Knight Ridder in Washington. *South China Morning Post*, 24 June 2002, 13.

Diet, nutrition and the prevention of chronic diseases: report of a Joint WHO/FAO Expert Consultation. Geneva, WHO, 2003 (WHO Technical Report Series No. 916):61.

Elliot A. US food industry ensures that consumers are not told to eat less. *British medical journal*, 2003, 327:1067.

Reuters Health Information 2004. US. drug sales $216.4 billion in 2003 – IMS report
http://www.medscape.com/viewarticle/469471?mpid=25157

American Heart Association. *Heart disease and stroke statistics – 2004 update*. Dallas, American Heart Association, 2003, Chapter 12:42.

National Institute of Neurological Disorders and Stroke. *Questions and answers about stroke*
http://www.ninds.nih.gov/health_and_medical/pubs/stroke_backgrounder.htm

United Kingdom
Vlad I. Obesity costs UK economy £2 bn a year. *British medical journal*, 2003, 327:1308.

Wise J. News: New clinical guidelines for stroke published. *British medical journal*, 2000, 320:823.

Netherlands
van Exel J, Koopmanschap MA, van Wijngaarden JDH, Scholte op Reimer WJM. Costs of stroke and stroke services: determinants of patient costs and a comparison of costs of regular care and care organised in stroke services. *Cost effectiveness and resource allocation*, 2003, 1:2
http://www.resource-allocation.com/content/1/1/2

Polder JJ, Meerding WJ, Koopmanschap MA, Bonneux L, van der Maas PJ. *Cost of illness in the Netherlands 1994*. Rotterdam, Instituut Maatschappelijke Gezondheidszorg [Institute for Medical Technology Assessment], Erasmus University, 1997
http://www.rivm.nl/kostenvanziekten/site_en/index.htm (in Dutch)

Evers SMAA, Struijs JN, Ament AJHA, van Genugten MLL, Jager JC, van den Bos GAM. *The disease impact, health care management, and costs of stroke in the Netherlands*. Bilthoven, National Institute for Public Health and the Environment (RIVM), 2002 (Report 282701001/2002).

Singapore
Venketasubramanian N, Yin A. Hospital costs for stroke care in Singapore. *Cerebrovascular diseases*, 2000, 10:320–326.

Price of weekly dose of medication
WHO cardiovascular Disease Programme. *Pilot survey on cost of cardiovascular drugs 2003* (unpublished data).

The cost of risk factors
Liu K, Daviglus ML, Yan LJ, Garside DB, Greenland P, Manheim LM, Dyer AR, Stamler J. Cardiovascular disease (CVD) risk factor status earlier in adulthood and cumulative health care costs from age 65 to the point of death. *Circulation*, 2004, 108:IV–722.

Lifetime costs of coronary heart disease
Klever-Deichert G, Hinzpeter B, Hunsche E, Lauterbach KW. *Zeitschrift für Kardiologie*, 1999, 88:991–1000.

Expenditure on cardiovascular medications
Dickson M, Jacobzone S. Pharmaceutical use and expenditure for cardiovascular disease and stroke: a study of 12 OECD countries. Paris, Organisation for Economic Co-operation and Development, 2003 (OECD Health working papers, DELSA/ELSA/WD/HEA(2003)1), Table 1.

Wow: Aspirin
Ebrahim S. Cost-effectiveness of stroke prevention. *British medical bulletin*, 2000, 56:557–570.

PART 4 ACTION

18 Research

Map: CVD research publications; Regional research

Mendis S, Yach D, Bengoa R, Narvaez D, Zhang X. Research gap in cardiovascular disease in developing countries. *Lancet*, 2003, 361:2246–2247.

Clinical trials

Search by authors, 24 February 2004.

Research funding by the National Institute of Health in the USA

United States Department of Health and Human Services. National Institutes of Health. *Estimates of funding for various diseases, conditions, research areas* http://www.nih.gov/news/fundingresearchareas.htm

Wow: United Kingdom

Rothwell PM. The high cost of not funding stroke research: a comparison with heart disease and cancer. *Lancet*, 2001, 357(9268):1612–1616 (review).

Bennett R, Burden S. UK funding for stroke research. *Lancet*, 2001, 358:1275 (correspondence).

Clipboard

Mendis S, Yach D, Bengoa R, Narvaez D, Zhang X. Research gap in cardiovascular disease in developing countries. *Lancet*, 2003, 361:2246–2247.

WHO. *The World Health Report 1999: Making a difference*. Geneva, WHO, 1999, Annex Table 3:108

Text

Baris E, Waverley Brigden L, Prindiville J, da Costa e Silva VL, Hatai C, Chandiwana S. Research priorities for tobacco control in developing countries: a regional approach to a global consultative process. *Tobacco control*, 2000, 9:217–23.

Tunstall-Pedoe H, ed. *MONICA monograph and multimedia sourcebook*. Prepared by Tunstall-Pedoe H, Kuulasmaa K, Tolonen H, Davidson M, Mendis S with 64 other contributors for The WHO MONICA Project. Geneva, WHO, 2003.

20 Prevention: personal choices and actions

Personal choices in lifestyles and behaviour; Personal actions for safeguarding cardiovascular health

Bulletin of the WHO, 1999.

Young people

Kavey RW, Daniels SR, Lauer RM, Atkins DL, Hayman LL, Taubert K. American Heart Association guidelines for primary prevention of atherosclerotic cardiovascular disease beginning in childhood. *Circulation*, 2003, 107:1562.

Eat fruit and cereals

Pereira MA, O'Reilly E, Augustsson K et al. Dietary fiber and risk of coronary heart disease. A pooled analysis of cohort studies. *Archives of internal medicine*, 2004, 164:370–376 http://archinte.ama-assn.org/cgi/content/abstract/164/4/370

The benefits of stopping smoking

American Lung Association. When smokers quit, within twenty minutes of smoking that last cigarette the body begins a series of changes http://www.lungusa.org/tobacco/quit_ben.html

Wow: USA; Clipboard: Burning calories

New "food pyramid" to address obesity epidemic. Reuters Health Information 2004 http://www.lifetimefitness.com/health_info/index.cfm?strWebAction=health_article&intArticleId=1384

Wow: Japan

Schnirring L. Can exercise gadgets motivate patients? *The physician and sportsmedicine*, news briefs, 2001, 29(1) http://www.physsportsmed.com/issues/2001/01_01/news.htm

Wow: Compared with less active…

HeartBytes. Reduce heart disease risk: encourage and prescribe exercise for your patients. *Medscape cardiology*, 2004, 8(1) http://www.medscape.com/viewarticle/470115?mpid=25341

Wow: People with low fitness...
Carnethon MR, Gidding SS, Nehgme R, Sidney S, Jacobs DR Jr, Liu K. Cardiorespiratory fitness in young adulthood and the development of cardiovascular disease risk factors. *Journal of the American Medical Association*, 2003, 290(23):3092–100.

Clipboard: For people with diabetes...
Standards of medical care in diabetes. *Diabetes care*, 2004, 27 (Suppl 1):S15–35.

Bilous R. Blood pressure control in type 2 diabetes – what does the United Kingdom Prospective Diabetes Study (PDS) tell us? *Nephrology dialysis and transplantation*, 1999, 14:2562–2564.

Clipboard: Reducing salt intake...
He FJ, MacGregor GA. How far should salt intake be reduced? *Hypertension*, 2003, 42(6):1093–9.

Text
O'Keefe JH Jr, Cordain L. Cardiovascular disease resulting from a diet and lifestyle at odds with our Paleolithic genome: how to become a 21st-century hunter-gatherer. *Mayo Clinics proceedings*, 2004, 79:101–108.

Carlsson CM, Stein JH. Cardiovascular disease and the aging woman: overcoming barriers to lifestyle changes. *Current women's health report*, 2002, 2:366–372.

21 Prevention: population and systems approaches

Noncommunicable disease prevention and control; Availability of equipment; Medical professionals; Antihypertensive drugs
Alwan A, Maclean D, Mandil A. *Assessment of national capacity for noncommunicable disease prevention and control; the report of a global survey*. Geneva, WHO, 2001.

Use of medications in stroke and coronary heart disease
Gaps in secondary prevention of myocardial infarction and stroke: WHO study on Prevention of REcurrences of Myocardial Infarction and StrokE (WHO-PREMISE) in low and middle income countries. WHO-PREMISE (Phase I) Study Group.

Wows: Finland; Japan; New Zealand; Mauritius
World Health Report 2002: reducing risks, promoting healthy life. Cardiovascular death and disability can be reduced more than 50%. Press Release WHO/83. 17 October 2002:6.

Clipboard
Institute of Medicine. *Crossing the quality chasm: a new health system for the 21st Century*. Washington, DC, National Academy Press, 2001
http://books.nap.edu/books/0309072808/html/1.html#pagetop

Text
Mendis S. Role of governments in improving prevention of cardiovascular disease. *Global Symposium on Cardiovascular Prevention, Marbella, Spain*, 11–13 April 2003.

Salim Y. Two decades of progress in preventing vascular disease. *Lancet*, 2002, 360
http://www.thelancet.com/journal/vol360/iss9326/full/llan.360.9326.editorial_and_review.21674.1

22 Health education

Map: World Heart Day
World Heart Federation. *World Heart Day*
http://www.worldheartday.com/news/news.asp?Page=HeartNews#

World Heart Day: themes; activities; Evaluation of
World Heart Day, A World Heart Federation enterprise promoting the prevention of heart disease and stroke across the world. *Circulation*, 2003, 108:1038–1040.

Grizeau-Clemens D. *Evaluation of 2001 World Heart Day coverage*. World Heart Federation, 2003.

Giving up smoking: International Quit and Win
Vartiainen ER, Project Manager, International Quit&Win, personal communication, 20 January 2004.

23 Policies and legislation

Map: Smoke-free workplaces
Shafey O, Dolwick S, Guindon GE, eds. *Tobacco control country profiles 2003*. Atlanta, GA, American Cancer Society, WHO, International Union Against Cancer, 2003.

Cardiovascular disease plans worldwide; Legislation
Policy data from: WHO. Capacity for NCD prevention and control survey 2001. *Assessment of national capacity for noncommunicable disease prevention and control. The report of a global survey*. Geneva, WHO, 2001.

Wow: 2002 USA
Sargent RP, Shepard RM, Glantz SA. Reduced incidence of admissions for myocardial infarction associated with public smoking ban: before and after study. *British medical journal*, 2004, 328:977–980.

24 Treatment

Cardiac rehabilitation; Patients reaching blood pressure and blood cholesterol goals during treatment
EUROASPIRE II Study Group (2001). Lifestyle and risk factor management and use of drug therapies in coronary patients from 15 countries. Principal results from EUROASPIRE II Euro Heart Survey Programme. *European heart journal*, 2001, 22:554–572.

Simple secondary prevention medication treatments
Yusuf S. Two decades of progress in preventing vascular disease. *Lancet*, 2002, 360:2–3 http://www.thelancet.com

Diabetes treatment
Ustun TB, Chatterji S, Mechbal A, Murray CJL, WHS Collaborating Groups. *The World Health Surveys in Health Systems Performance Assessment: debates, methods and empiricism*. Murray CJL and Evans DB, eds, Geneva, WHO, 2003.

Trends in cardiovascular operations and procedures in the USA
American Heart Association. *Heart disease and stroke statistics – 2004 update*. Dallas, American Heart Association, 2003.

Wow: Proportion of people…
Mensah GA. The global burden of hypertension: good news and bad news. *Cardiology clinics*, 2002, 20(2):181–185

Wolf-Maier K, Cooper RS, Banegas JR et al. Hypertension prevalence and blood pressure levels in 6 European countries, Canada, and the United States. *Journal of the American Medical Association*, 2003, 289(18):2363–2369.

Wow: In the USA, only 24%…
Ford ES, Mokdad AH, Giles WH, Mensah GA. Serum total cholesterol concentrations and awareness, treatment, and control of hypercholesterolemia among US adults: findings from the National Health and Nutrition Examination Survey, 1999 to 2000. *Circulation*, 2003, 107(17):2185–2189.

Text
Gunn J, Crossman D, Grech ED, Cumberland D. New developments in percutaneous coronary intervention. *British medical journal*, 2003, 327(7407):150–153.

Mensah GA. Eliminating health disparities: the time for action is now. *Ethnicity and disease*, 2002, 12(1):3–7.

PART 5 THE FUTURE AND THE PAST

25 Future

DALYs; Deaths
WHO (2004). Unpublished projections from 2000 baseline, prepared for *The World Health Report 2002*, using projection methods developed by Murray CJL, Lopez AD. *The global burden of disease*. Boston, Harvard School of Public Health, 1996, Chapter 7:325–395.

Risk factors

Mackay J, Eriksen M. *The tobacco atlas.* Geneva, WHO, 2002:90–91.

Wild S, Roglic G, Green A, Sicree R, King H. Global prevalence of diabetes. Estimates for the year 2000 and projections for 2030. *Diabetes care*, 2004, 27:1047–1053.

Amos AF, McCarty DJ, Zimmet P. The rising global burden of diabetes and its complications: estimates and projections to the year 2010. *Diabetes medicine*, 1997, 14 (Suppl 5):S1–S5.

Collins R, Clinical Trial Service Unit, University of Oxford, England, personal communication, 6 January 2004.

Economic costs

REUTERS in Washington. United States: US obesity weighs heavy on health costs. *South China Morning Post*, 10 March 2004, A12 (study by Rand Corporation).

Action

Guttmacher AE, Collins FS. Genomic medicine: a primer. *New England journal of medicine*, 2002, 347:1512–1550.

Wolf CR, Smith G, Smith RL. Science, medicine, and the future: pharmacogenetics. *British medical journal*, 2000, 320:987–990.

Mackay J, Eriksen M. *The tobacco atlas.* Geneva, WHO, 2002:90–91.

Treatment

Pearson I. *Atlas of the future.* New York, Macmillan, 1998:32–33.

American Federation for Aging Research. *What is the future of heart disease research likely to tell us?* http://www.infoaging.org/d-heart-11-future.html

Roden DM. Cardiovascular pharmacogenomics. *Circulation*, 2003, 108:3071–3074.

Crossman D. Science, medicine, and the future. The future of the management of ischaemic heart disease. *British medical journal*, 1997, 314:356–359.

Wald NJ, Law MR. A strategy to reduce cardiovascular disease by more than 80%. *British medical journal*, 2003, 326:1419.

Collins R, Clinical Trial Service Unit, University of Oxford, England, personal communication, 6 January 2004.

Text

Rodgers A, Lawes C, MacMahon S. Reducing the global burden of blood pressure-related cardiovascular disease. *Hypertension*, 2000, 18(1 Suppl):S3–6.

Lawes CM, Bennett DA, Feigin VL, Rodgers A. Blood pressure and stroke: an overview of published reviews. *Stroke*, 2004, 35(3):776–85.

Milestones in knowledge of heart and vascular disorders

Major sources

Baddarni K. *Historic aspects of cardiology* http://www.geocities.com/baddarni/Cardiology-History.html

Weisse AB. *Heart to heart: the twentieth century battle against cardiac disease: an oral history*. London, USA, Rutgers University Press, 2002.

Stamler J. *Lectures on preventive cardiology*. New York, Grune & Stratton, 1967 (cited in Vance DE, van den Bosch H. Cholesterol in the year 2000. *Biochemica et biophysica acta*, 2000, 1529:1–8

Wan S, Yim APC. The evolution of cardiovascular surgery in China. *Annals of thoracic surgery*, 2003, 76:2147–55.

A timeline of milestones from The Framingham Heart Study http://www.framingham.com/heart/timeline.htm

Schooler C, Farquhar JW, Fortmann SP, Flora JA. Synthesis of findings and issues from community prevention trials. *Annals of epidemiology*, 1997, S7:S54–68.

World Health Organization

http://www.who.int

Cardiovascular disease:
http://www5.who.int/cardiovascular-diseases/
Diabetes:
http://www.who.int/health_topics/diabetes_mellitus/en/
Diet:
http://www.who.int/health_topics/diet/en/
Nutrition:
http://www.who.int/health_topics/nutrition/en/
Obesity:
http://www.who.int/health_topics/obesity/en/
Public Health Surveillance:
http://www.who.int/health_topics/public_health_surveillance/en/
Tobacco Free Initiative:
http://www.who.int/tobacco/en/

Centers for Disease Control and Prevention, USA

http://www.cdc.gov/

Cardiovascular Health Program:
http://www.cdc.gov/cvh/
Nutrition and Physical Activity Program:
http://www.cdc.gov/nccdphp/dnpa/
Tobacco Program:
http://www.cdc.gov/tobacco/
Diabetes Program:
http://www.cdc.gov/diabetes/
Laboratory Sciences Program:
http://www.cdc.gov/nceh/dls/programs.htm
Office of Global Health:
http://www.cdc.gov/ogh/
Behavioral Risk Factor Surveillance System:
http://www.cdc.gov/brfss
National Center for Health Statistics:
http://www.cdc.gov/nchs

International and Regional Organisations

Asian Society for Cardiovascular Surgery:
http://www.ascvs.org/
Association for European Paediatric Cardiology/Association
Européenne pour la Cardiologie Pédiatrique:
http://www.aepc.org/home.htm
Brain Aneurysm Foundation:
http://www.bafound.org
Cairdes: http://www.cairdes.com
CardioStart International Inc:
http://www.cardiostart.com/
Cardiothoracic Surgery Network:
http://www.ctsnet.org/
Chain of Hope: http://www.chainofhope.org
Children's HeartLink:
http://www.childrensheartlink.org/
Children's Hearts: http://www.childrenshearts.org.uk
Clearinghouse for Tobacco Control (South East Asia):
http://www.prn2.usm.my/pages/about.asp
Cœurs pour Tous (Hearts for All):
http://www.cptg.ch/fr/start.htm
Congenital Heart Information Network:
http://www.tchin.org/

Congress of Neurological Surgeons:
http://www.neurosurgeon.org
Consortium for Southeastern Hypertension Control (COSEHC):
http://www.cosehc.org/
East Meets West: http://www.eastmeetswest.org
Eastern Mediterranean Network on Heart Health, (EMNHH):
http://emnhh.homestead.com/files/index.htm
The Endocrine Society: http://www.endo-society.org/
European Association for Cardiothoracic Surgery:
http://www.eacts.org/
European Heart Institute:
http://www.european-academy.at
European Heart Network:
http://www.ehnheart.org/index2.asp
EMASH European Medical Association on Smoking and Health:
http://emash.globalink.org/
ENSH European Network for Smoke-free Hospitals:
http://ensh.free.fr/
ENSP European Network for Smoking Prevention:
http://www.ensp.org
European Network of Young People and Tobacco:
http://www.ktl.fi/enypat/
European Network of Quitlines:
http://www.quitlines-conference.com/
European Society for Noninvasive Cardiovascular Dynamics:
http://www2.mf.uni-lj.si/~esnicvd/
European Society of Cardiology:
http://www.escardio.org/
European Society of Hypertension:
http://www.eshonline.org/
European Stroke Initiative:
http://www.eusi-stroke.com/index.shtml
European Union of Non-smokers:
http://www.globalink.org/tobacco/docs/eu-docs/uene.htm
Framework Convention Alliance (FCA):
http://www.fctc.org/
G8 Telematics Heart Health Project:
http://www.med.mun.ca/g8hearthealth/
Gift of Life International Inc.:
http://www.giftoflifeinternational.org/
Global Connection International:
http://www.gciworld.org
Global Cardiovascular Infobase (in English and Spanish):
http://www.cvdinfobase.ca/
Global Healing: http://www.globalhealing.org
Global Health Information Network:
http://www.healthnet.org/
Global Partnerships for Tobacco Control:
http://www.essentialaction.org/tobacco/
Globalink, UICC International Union against Cancer:
http://www.globalink.org/
Healing the Children:
http://www.healingchildren.org
Heart Care International:
http://www.heartcareintl.org
HeartGift Foundation:
http://www.heartgift.org/index.html
The Heart of a Child Foundation – Little Hearts on the Mend:
http://www.littleheartsonthemend.org
Heart-to-Heart International:
http://www.hearttoheart.org/

Heart-to-Heart International Children's Medical Alliance:
http://www.heart-2-heart.org/
Initiative for Cardiovascular Health Research in Developing Countries:
http://www.globalforumhealth.org/pages/index.asp?
ThePage=page1_000500040001_1.htm&Nav=000500040001
InterAmerican Heart Foundation:
http://www.interamericanheart.org
InterAmerican Society of Cardiology (in Spanish and English):
http://www.soinca.org
Inter-American Society of Hypertension:
http://org.umc.edu/iash/homepage.htm:
http://www.musc.edu/iash/generale.htm
International Academy of Cardiology:
http://www.cardiologyonline.com/
International Agency on Tobacco and Health (IATH):
Email: admin@iath.org
International Atherosclerosis Society:
http://www.athero.org/
International Children's Heart Foundation:
http://www.ichf.org/
International Children's Heart Fund:
http://www.ichfund.org/
International Diabetes Federation:
http://www.idf.org/
International Diabetes Institute, Australia:
http://www.diabetes.com.au/home.htm
International Federation of Sports Medicine:
http://www.fims.org/
International Hospital for Children (IHC):
http://www.healachild.org
International Network of Women against Tobacco (INWAT):
http://www.inwat.org/
International Network towards Smoke-Free Hospitals (INTSH):
http://intsh.globalink.org/
International Non Governmental Coalition against Tobacco (INGCAT):
http://www.ingcat.org/
International Obesity Task Force:
http://www.iotf.org/
International Pediatric Hypertension Association:
http://www.pediatrichypertension.org/
International Society for Adult Congenital Cardiac Disease:
http://www.isaccd.org/
International Society for Aging and Physical Activity:
http://www.isapa.org/
International Society for Cardiovascular Surgery:
http://www.vascsurg.org/doc/1576.html##.htm
International Society for Heart Research:
http://www.ishrworld.org/
International Society for Heart & Lung Transplantation:
http://www.ishlt.org/
International Society for Minimally Invasive Cardiac Surgery:
http://www.ismics.org/
International Society for the Prevention of Tobacco Induced Diseases
(PTID): http://www.ptid.org
International Society of Cardiovascular Ultrasound:
http://www.iscu.org/
International Society of Hypertension:
http://www.hypertension2004.com.br/
International Society of Nephrology:
http://www.isn-online.org/
International Society on Hypertension in Blacks (ISHIB):
http://www.ishib.org/main/ishib_open.htm
International Stroke Society:
http://www.internationalstroke.org/index.php
International Task Force for the Prevention of Coronary Heart Disease:
http://www.chd-taskforce.de/

International Tobacco Evidence Network (ITEN):
http://www.tobaccoevidence.net/
The Internet Stroke Center:
http://www.strokecenter.org/pat/organizations.htm
Legacy Foundation, tobacco document site:
http://legacy.library.ucsf.edu/cgi/b/bib/bib-idx?g=tob
Mediterranean Stroke Society:
http://www.hsanmartino.liguria.it/cictus/med.htm
OTAF L'Observatoire du Tabac en Afrique Francophone:
http://otaf.globalink.org/
Physicians for Peace: http://www.physiciansforpeace.org
ProCOR: Conference on Cardiovascular Health:
http://www.procor.org/
Project Hope: http://www.projecthope.org
Project Kids Worldwide:
http://www.projectkidsworldwide.org
Project Open Hearts: http://www.poh.org
Repace's site, especially on passive smoking (Jim Repace):
http://www.repace.com/
Save A Child's Heart Foundation:
http://www.saveachildsheart.com
Society for Research on Nicotine and Tobacco (SRNT):
http://www.srnt.org/
Smokescreen Action Network:
http://www.smokescreen.org
Southeast Asian Tobacco Control Alliance:
http://www.tobaccofreeasia.net/
Stroke Awareness for Everyone:
http://www.strokesafe.org/
Stroke Clubs International:
Email: strokeclub@aol.com
Stroke Net:
http://www.strokenet.info/resources/stroke/internationalsites.htm
Surgeons of Hope Foundation:
http://www.surgeonsofhope.org
Tobacco.org: http://www.tobacco.org
Tobacco Control journal:
http://www.tobaccocontrol.com
Tobacco Control Resource Center/Tobacco Products Liability Project
(TCRC/TPLP): http://tobacco.neu.edu/
TCRC Tobacco Control Resource Centre, BMA, UK:
http://www.tobacco-control.org/
Tobacco Control Supersite:
http://www.health.usyd.edu.au/tobacco/
Tobacco Documents Online (TDO, Smokescreen:
http://www.tobaccodocuments.org
Tobaccopedia:
http://TobaccoPedia.org
Treatobacco Database & Educational Resource for Treatment of
Tobacco Dependence:
http://www.treatobacco.net/
World Federation of Neurology:
http://www.wfneurology.org/
World Heart Federation:
http://www.worldheart.org/
World Heart Foundation:
http://www.world-heart.org/
World Hypertension League:
http://www.mco.edu/org/whl/
World Kidney Foundation:
http://www.worldkidneyfund.org/
World Medical Association:
http://www.wma.net/